DRUGS AND PREGNANCY

The Effects of Nonmedical Use of Drugs
on Pregnancy, Childbirth, and Neonates

Edited by

Patricia Ferguson, M.L.S.
Documentation Associates

Thomas Lennox, M.L.S.
Documentation Associates

and

Dan J. Lettieri, Ph.D.
Division of Research
Behavioral and Social Sciences Branch
National Institute on Drug Abuse

November 1974

National Institute on Drug Abuse
11400 Rockville Pike
Rockville, Maryland 20852

For sale by the Superintendent of Documents, U.S. Government Printing Office, Washington, D.C. 20402

This volume, part of a Research Issues Series, was prepared for the National Institute on Drug Abuse by Documentation Associates, Box 25892, Los Angeles, California, under Contract Number HSM-42-73-222.

DHEW Publication No. (ADM) 75-187
Printed 1975

FOREWORD

The issues of drug use and abuse have generated many volumes of words, all written in an attempt to explain the "problem" and suggest the "solution." Data have been generated by researchers from many disciplines, each looking at a particular aspect of an issue. The present booklet is one of a new series intended to aid researchers who find it difficult to find the time to scan, let alone read all the information which exists and which continues to be published daily in their area of interest. An attempt has been made to focus predominantly on empirical research findings and major theoretical approaches.

Included in volumes 1 through 7 of the series are summaries of the major research findings of the last 15 years, formulated and detailed to provide the reader with the purpose, methodology, findings and conclusions of previous studies done in the topic area. Each topic was chosen because it represented a challenging issue of current interest to the research community. As additional issues are identified, the relevant research will be published as part of this series.

Several of the volumes in the series represent a departure from the above description. These also represent challenging issues, and issues of current interest; they are, however, virtually unexplored areas which have received little attention from the research world. For example, the subjects of drugs and the visual arts, science fiction, and fiction--aspects of contemporary life which impact on all of us--are explored here by writers who have been deeply involved in those fields. Their content is perhaps provocative, and certainly stimulating.

The Research Issues series is a group project of staff members of the National Institute on Drug Abuse, Division of Research, Behavioral and Social Sciences Branch. Special thanks are due to the continued guidance and support of Dr. Louise Richards and Dr. Norman Krasnegor. Selection of articles for inclusion was greatly aided by the suggestions of a peer review group, researchers themselves, each of whom reviewed a topic of particular interest. It is my pleasure to acknowledge their contribution to the project here.

Dan J. Lettieri, Ph.D.
Project Officer
National Institute on Drug Abuse

iii

ACKNOWLEDGMENTS

A bibliographic project such as this necessarily involved a great number of people, all of whom contributed their own particular talent. Many worked on more than one phase of the project. Many more are not named here--their help and advice was instrumental in shaping and defining the series and the individual topics. It is important, however, to distinguish between the members of the peer review group who were instrumental in the initial selection of the articles to be included and abstracted, and the members of the abstracting team who bear sole responsibility for the final format and content of the abstract of each research paper included in this volume.

Peer Review Group

Michael Baden, M.D.
John Ball, Ph.D.
Richard Blum, Ph.D.
Carl Chambers, Ph.D.
Joel Fort, Ph.D.
George Gay, M.D.
Gilbert Geis, Ph.D.
Louis Gottschalk, M.D.
Raymond Harbison, Ph.D.
Richard Jessor, Ph.D.
Denise Kandel, Ph.D.
Gerald Kline, Ph.D.
Norman Krasnegor, Ph.D.

Irving Lukoff, Ph.D.
William McGlothlin, Ph.D.
David Nurco, D.S.W.
Stephen Pittel, Ph.D.
Louise Richards, Ph.D.
Alex Richman, M.D.
Charles Rohrs, M.D.
Elaine Schwartz, Ph.D.
Saul Sells, Ph.D.
Irving Soloway, Ph.D.
Forrest Tennant, M.D.
Dan Waldorf, M.A.

The Abstracting Team consisted of: Greg Austin; David Harris; Susan Hope; Diane Kovacs; Cynthia Lundquist; Marianne Moerman; Roger Owens and Carolee Rosser.

PREFACE

An extensive and comprehensive literature search was carried out to identify materials for inclusion in the Research Issues series. Major clearinghouses, data bases, library collections, and previous bibliographies were searched, either through an automated system or manually. Special efforts were made to correspond with organizations, institutions and individuals who might have relevant materials. Current issues of newsletters and journals were scanned throughout the project. A selective list of the sources accessed includes:

National Clearinghouse for Drug Abuse Information (NCDAI)

NCDAI: Report Series, Selected Reference Series

Drug Abuse Current Awareness System (DACAS)

SPEED: The Current Index to Drug Abuse Literature

Grassroots

Addiction Research Foundation, Bibliographies

Drug Dependence

Psychological Abstracts (PASAR)

Sociological Abstracts

Dissertation Abstracts

Index Medicus (MEDLINE)

Addiction: Bioresearch Today

Research in Education (ERIC: RIE)

Public Affairs Information Service (PAIS)

Monthly Catalog of U.S. Government Documents

Music Index

Art Index

Guide to the Performing Arts

Reader's Guide to Periodical Literature

The criteria for selection of documents were drawn up by a consultant group of drug researchers working with the contractor and representatives of the National Institute on Drug Abuse. For inclusion a study had to meet the following general criteria:

(1)   empirical research studies with findings pertinent to the particular topic, or major theoretical approaches to the study of that topic

(2)   published between January 1958 and January 1974, preferably in the professional literature, with the exception of certain older "classics" which merited inclusion and unpublished dissertations

(3)   English language; however, since the focus was on American drug issues, those English language materials which dealt with aspects of drug use encountered largely in other countries were excluded.

After a first review of citations and annotations, to weed out obviously irrelevant materials, the body of collected literature was subjected to two reviews: one to ensure that materials met the selection criteria, and a second by a peer review group to ensure that studies representative of the universe were included.

TABLE OF CONTENTS

Page

I.   OVERVIEWS.. 1

    I. 01   Genetics...................................... 2

    I. 02   Epidemiology................................. 5

    I. 04   Effects of Drugs on Neonates 10

II.   LSD 29

    II. 01   Literature Reviews.......................... 30

    II. 05   Chromosome Studies 40

    II. 09   Teratogenesis Studies 51

III. HEROIN 57

    III. 01   Mother and Child......................... 58

    III. 06   Characteristics of Neonates Born to Heroin Users.. 71

    III. 14   Neonatal Withdrawal Management................. 93

IV.   METHADONE..101

V.   METHADONE AND HEROIN: COMPARATIVE STUDIES......117

VI.   SELECTED ANNOTATED STUDIES 131

I.   OVERVIEWS

Falek, Arthur, and Einstein, Stanley. Genetics and drug abuse:
A primer for workers in the field. Drug Forum, 2(4):377-394.
Summer, 1973. (12 references).

SUMMARY

This report described some basic information about human genetics with particular attention to the effects of drugs of abuse on
human chromosomes. Relevant findings were presented about
human chromosomes from both somatic and reproductive cells
as well as a summary of the evidence about the kinds, frequencies,
and implications of the observed cytogenetic damage due to drugs
of abuse. The limitations and directions of present research investigations were discussed.

The multi-generation effects of mutants which produce mild alterations are of significance in investigating the genetic consequences
of drug abuse. The difficulties in evaluating the Drosophila data,
based as it is on carefully designed, controlled mating experiments, indicate that it would not be possible to measure such
minimal changes in the human population. However, the Drosophila findings suggest that similar damage is occurring in man.

While controlled studies which would meet rigid scientific require-
ments are not possible with persons taking illicit drugs, one feasible method to predict some possible genetic consequences of
drug abuse is that of cytogenetic (chromosome) examination. One
important group to investigate for chromosome damage would be
those at high risk in the newborn population -- infants of parents
reporting drug abuse. A general examination of these infants
should also be conducted for any sign of congenital defects, and
the infants should be compared to a control group. It is important
that those who are concerned with drug misuse understand the
potential as well as the limits of cytogenetic studies. Chromosome studies will only reveal gross kinds of aberrations.

While banding techniques have not yet been incorporated into
cytogenetic studies of patients in drug abuse programs, available
evidence indicates that some of these patients have a population
of cells with damaged chromosomes. The damage observed does
not indicate the amount or frequency of use required to initiate or
maintain this damage. In both drug abusers and control subjects
single and double chromatid gaps, as well as chromatid breaks,

have been observed. In addition to chromatid gaps and breaks, patients in a multiple drug population revealed dicentric chromosomes and exchange figures as well as ring chromosomes. Not all multiple drug patients seem to respond cytogenetically to drug ingestion in the same way. In certain individuals, as a consequence of drug ingestion, synthesized chromosomes appear to break in response to the trauma of the technical procedures which occur in the culture.

Most in vivo studies with patients on drugs of abuse have not as yet met the rigid criteria essential to high scientific standards. With regard to in vivo studies with LSD, problems in design have included small sample size, exposure of patients and controls to other drugs, limited data in both groups with regard to radiation therapy, and viral infections immediately prior to cytogenetic study. In almost all instances control subjects for comparison with the patient population have been matched in only the most minimal fashion. In vitro studies also require special attention. Such studies may show no damage because the drug or chemical in question does not penetrate into the cell. Metabolic alterations may be affected by pH and by other biochemical parameters which control the accessibility and activity of the drug or its products in the cells of the body. These alterations are not included for study in most programs when the drugs are introduced directly into the culture. In addition to in vivo and in vitro human cytogenetic studies, a variety of other program designs have been employed utilizing chromosome evaluation, dominant lethal assays and microbial studies to determine mutagenicity. For these programs testing has been conducted in animals other than man.

At the present time there is no reliable method for the early detection of a genetic catastrophe introduced by new chemicals and drugs. Our methods only permit indirect experimental genetic studies which will not detect a rapid increase in damage to the human gene pool which is not anticipated; current test procedures are beset with many difficulties inherent in any attempt to extrapolate plant, bacterial, and other animal test data to man, with regard to specificity of response, correlation between types of damage, and dose-effect relationships.

There are individual differences in human cytogenetic response to drugs, and in some individuals multiple drug use appears to have a synergistic effect (cooperative interaction) which appears to result in an increased frequency of chromosome fragility. Obviously there is a need to develop more accurate methods to evaluate the potential of all drugs, including drugs of abuse, and researchers are suggesting a variety of tests, although all test systems at present contain methodological difficulties.

3

This could be done even if their concentrations were so low that any direct test on a person or his descendants would not be powerful enough to detect the effect.

CONCLUSIONS

Somatic cytogenetic studies are now being done, but better criteria are needed for distinguishing those types of aberrations that are correlated with genetic damage that is transmitted to future generations. Effective methods for detecting somatic gene mutations do not appear to be beyond present technology. A search for phenotypic abnormalities in new-born children of drug users, combined with a search for teratogenic effects might be economically feasible as well as highly productive.

Crow, J.F. Epidemiological surveillance of human populations
for mutational hazards. In: Epstein, Samuel S., ed. Drugs of
Abuse, Their Genetic and Other Chronic Nonpsychiatric Hazards.
Cambridge, Mass.: MIT Press, 1971. pp. 196-200. (5 references)

SUMMARY

The author discussed several methods for population monitoring
which seemed to be most promising. A monitoring system must
be relevant, prompt, sensitive, broad, organized, and economically feasible. Somatic cell indicators are needed whereby the
individual cell, rather than the person, is the unit of observation.

A need exists for better ways of identifying in somatic cells those
kinds of chromosomal events that indicate transmittable genetic
damage. One possibility would be to concentrate specifically on
chromosome breaks of particular kinds. High research priority
was suggested for a systematic study of the correlation among
particular kinds of cytological configurations in somatic cells of
the parent, and genetic damage in the descendants.

Also needed are in vivo tests for somatic point mutations. Early
work was done by Atwood with human red blood cell antigens.
The author felt it should be possible to find systems that detect
both forward and reverse mutations.

New-born infants of drug-using parents could possibly provide
direct evidence of genetic change. Perhaps the best procedure
would be an examination of each new-born infant of drug-using
parents for any sign of congenital defect. This could be combined
with a similar program for detection of teratogens. The discov-
ery of any phenotype that was previously rare or absent is a danger signal. It could also be valuable to examine the history of
children with congenital anomalies and mental retardation.

Various body measurements could be used, such as Lederberg's
suggestion that minor asymmetries might be indicators of an
imbalance caused by mutation. A lowered IQ is a particularly
sensitive indicator that something has gone wrong.

Another possible monitoring system would be to see if the blood
serum of drug users contained substances that were mutagenic in
other test systems. It may be discovered that there are mutagenic influences not explained by the drug itself. Such influences
might be determined by a highly efficient microbial test system.

Since the risk of damage from the level of the gene to that of clinically visible morphologic defects is not only of significance as a population problem for future generations, but is of immediate concern to the individual and his offspring, the development and evaluation of methods for study of the genetic aspects of drug abuse is important. It is the scientist's responsibility to develop these methods and the role of community leaders to take an active part in making use of this technical data for the benefit of the community.

Forfar, John O., and Nelson, Matilda M. Epidemiology of drugs
taken by pregnant women: Drugs that may affect the fetus
adversely. Clinical Pharmacology and Therapeutics, 14(4-Part 2):
632-642, July-August, 1973.

DRUG	Multi-Drug
SAMPLE SIZE	911
SAMPLE TYPE	Treatment (inpatient)
AGE	Not Specified
SEX	Female
ETHNICITY	Not Specified
GEOGRAPHICAL AREA	Edinburgh, Scotland
METHODOLOGY	Case Study
DATA COLLECTION INSTRUMENT	Interviews and Program/Clinic Statistics
DATE(S) CONDUCTED	Not Specified
NO. OF REFERENCES	37

SUMMARY

The epidemiology of drug consumption during pregnancy was
studied retrospectively in 911 randomly selected mothers. Structured interviews, as well as hospital and pharmacy records, were
used to ascertain the drugs used, the proportions of pregnant
women taking them, and the duration and timing of drug administration. Excluding iron, drugs were prescribed for 82% of women
during pregnancy, and the average number of drugs prescribed for
these women was 4. Self-medicated drugs were taken by 65% of
mothers, and the average number taken by these was 1. 5.

Some drugs tended to be administered early, some late, and some throughout pregnancy. A drug "consumption in pregnancy" factor was calculated so that the overall consumption of a drug could be measured and comparisons made of the consumption of one drug relative to another. Drugs that may carry a risk of teratogenicity if administered early in pregnancy are listed, as are those drugs that, if administered later, may adversely affect fetal or neonatal functioning.

METHODOLOGY

A study of drug consumption in pregnancy, and the relationship of this to congenital abnormalities, was carried out in Edinburgh. Information was obtained from 911 mothers shortly after delivery, by means of a structured interview carried out in each case by the same interviewer. Hospital records were examined, physicians involved were consulted, and prescription records were checked. A drug was accepted as being consumed only if there were two indications that it had been used. The mothers were randomly selected, with the exception that none had a child with a significant congenital malformation.

FINDINGS

Drugs conspicuous by their absence or infrequency of usage were steroids, antihypertensive drugs, anticoagulants, antithyroid drugs, thyroid, digitalis, ergot and ergotlike substances, insulin, muscle relaxants, and rigidity- and tremor-controlling drugs. Drugs taken were classified as "early pregnancy," "late pregnancy," or "throughout pregnancy" drugs, to designate what time during pregnancy drugs were administered.

Findings show that, excluding iron, drugs had been prescribed for 82% of the women during pregnancy, and the average number prescribed was 4. Self-medicated drugs were taken by 65% of the women, and the average number taken was 1.5. The proportion of mothers taking different categories of drugs ranged from 82% to 1.2%. The mean duration of drug therapy for the various categories of drugs ranged from 125 to 10 days. Fifty-seven percent of the women smoked, and only 12% abstained completely from alcohol.

Of the drugs prescribed for "medical" purposes, analgesics (especially aspirin) rated twice as high as any other category. Next came barbiturates, then antacids, diuretics, antiemetics, and drugs acting on the respiratory system. These were followed by the combined groups of antibiotics and sulfonamides, tranquilizers and hypnotics combined, antihistamines, and appetite suppressants.

8

CONCLUSIONS

Before attempting to identify those drugs that may affect the fetus adversely, the authors offered four points of caution:

1. Very little information is available about the effects of most drugs on the human fetus, and species differences may mean that many animal experiments are irrelevant.

2. An association between the consumption of a drug during pregnancy and an adverse effect on the fetus does not necessarily imply causation.

3. The degree of risk has to be taken into account, for each individual drug used.

4. Clinical indications for the usage of a drug have to be considered.

Possibly harmful drugs in pregnancy can be divided into 2 main groups: Those that have a teratogenic effect - essentially affecting the embryo in the first three months of pregnancy - and those that affect fetal function later in pregnancy, or the functions of the neonatal period. No drug used in therapy has shown the same teratogenic potency as thalidomide. It may be that many teratogenic effects of a lesser degree have still to be recognized. The authors include a table that lists those drugs in which there is a recognized association between administration early in pregnancy and teratogenic effects on the fetus.

Drugs with a possible slight teratogenic effect, if taken early in pregnancy, were mentioned: barbiturates, aspirin, plenytoin and dexamphetamine. Drugs possibly affecting the fetus late in pregnancy were seen to be : narcotics (if the mother is addicted), possibly inhalational and local anesthetics, barbiturates, and alcohol.

Brazelton, T. Berry. Effect of prenatal drugs on the behavior of
the neonate. American Journal of Psychiatry, 126(9):1261-1266,
March, 1970. (34 references).

SUMMARY

The author reviewed several studies dealing with the effects of
various drugs (taken prenatally) on newborn infants. Drugs which
are often medically prescribed for pregnant women included
progesterone (used to prevent abortion), codeine, tranquilizers, and
barbiturates.

Progesterone has been reported to cause an overmasculinization
of male infants (hypertrophy of penis and scrotum, exceptional
muscle development, irritability) and pseudomasculinization of
females (enlarged clitoris and neuromuscular tissue, and "mascu-
linized" behavior). Codeine was reported to cause withdrawal
symptoms similar to those seen in the infants of heroin or morphine-
addicted mothers.

Tranquilizers, commonly used as medication during labor, have
been shown to cause a delayed period of relative unresponsiveness
in newborn infants (including depressed motor activity and slow
heart and respiratory rates).

Barbiturates have been shown to compete with other substances in
an infant's system for detoxification. Also, the infant's midbrain
stores barbiturates at higher concentrations than blood level and
affects the CNS reactions and midbrain-mediated behavior for
up to a week after birth.

Meperidine and methazine were found to have transient effects on
the EEG's of 29 out of 33 infants.

Impaired sucking and breast feeding behavior have been noted as
the results of maternal medication, as confirmed by a delay in the
infant's weight gain. Inhaled anesthesia (type not noted) was found
to have relatively little effect on infants.

Acute alcohol withdrawal led to fever, alternating hyperirritability
and lethargy, and severe hyperbilirubinemia in the neonate.

Fetal abnormalities, chromosomal defects, and a high abortion
rate were noted in studies of infants whose mothers had ingested
LSD, but no behavioral analysis was done on the neonates.

Prenatal nutrition (particularly protein intake) was mentioned as an important factor in infant development.

CONCLUSIONS

The infant's phenotype is influenced initially by the intrauterine environment. His genotype may also be irreversibly affected during the critical period of early pregnancy when cellular development is rapid. The common use of depressant drugs during labor may have an adverse effect on the early mother-infant relationship and could possibly have lasting effects on their attachment.

Because of the important influence of the prenatal period on the infant, the author suggests that pediatricians and psychiatrists should work toward a more scientific and justified use of drugs and hormones in pregnancy (along with attention to the prenatal diet).

Sussman, Sidney. Narcotic and methamphetamine use during pregnancy: Effect on newborn infants. American Journal of Diseases of Children, 106(3):325-330, 1963.

DRUG	Multi-Drug
SAMPLE SIZE	23
SAMPLE TYPE	Parent-child; Treatment (inpatient)
AGE	23 Neonates
SEX	13 Male; 10 Female
ETHNICITY	12 White; 9 Black; 2 Other
GEOGRAPHICAL AREA	San Francisco, California
METHODOLOGY	Case Studies
DATA COLLECTION INSTRUMENT	Laboratory/Examination
DATE(S) CONDUCTED	1954-1962
NO. OF REFERENCES	14

SUMMARY

The study examined the effect upon newborn infants of narcotic and methamphetamine use by the mother during pregnancy. Nineteen addict mothers and their 12 premature and 11 full-term infants born at San Francisco General Hospital from 1954-1962 were studied. Most of the mothers were unmarried and did not have prenatal care. Diacetylmorphine (heroin) alone was used during 12 pregnancies; diacetylmorphine together with codeine in 3; codeine and barbiturates in 1; marijuana in 1; 4 took methamphetamine (methedrine); the drug was unknown in 1 case. Diacetylmorphine predominated prior to 1962, methamphetamine since. Five mothers showed signs of

recent narcotic use upon entry; five additional mothers had withdrawal symptoms during the post-partum period. Six infants were
breech births, 11 exhibited respiratory distress, 17 had withdrawal
symptoms. Swaddling and demand feeding controlled withdrawal
symptoms in most cases. Follow-up on 10 infants revealed normal
development in 9, and mental retardation in 1 case.

METHODOLOGY

Subjects for the study met at least one of three criteria: a history
of narcotic or methamphetamine use; withdrawal symptoms in the
mother during parturition or post-partum; withdrawal symptoms in
the infant. Data were tabulated for each case by drug, last pre-
delivery "fix," parturition type, onset and treatment of withdrawal
symptoms of infant, other symptoms, follow-up, sex, race and birth
weight. Table 1 presents the findings for 18 heroin cases; Table 2
for 4 methedrine cases. Since withdrawal symptoms in newborns
are often vague and apparently insignificant, a history of maternal
addiction or maternal withdrawal symptoms was used to assist in
substantiating diagnosis of neonatal addiction. Time of the mother's
last fix was correlated with onset of infant withdrawal symptoms,
and the association of withdrawal symptoms in mother and infant
analyzed. Follow-up information was collected on 9 addicted and 1
asymptomatic offspring.

FINDINGS

A predominance of central nervous system, gastrointestinal and
respiratory symptoms were observed in the narcotic addicted babies.
Most striking were convulsions, tremors, excessive irritability,
shrill crying, yawning and sneezing. Findings showed that absence
of maternal symptoms does not rule out diagnosis of newborn
addiction. Development of newborn withdrawal symptoms depends
on the maternal dose, the time interval between the last injection,
and delivery. A fix within one week of delivery was usually associated
with withdrawal symptoms in the infant; a fix prior to that was
usually asymptomatic. Mild withdrawal symptoms were found to be
manageable by swaddling, infrequent handling, demand feeding, and
attention to hydration. Results suggested that use of promethazine
and phenobarbital is ineffective.

CONCLUSIONS

Addiction in newborns is a reflection of addiction in women of childbearing age. Morphine use has given way to diacetylmorphine and
presently there is increased use of methamphetamine among addicts.
Methamphetamine does not cause addiction and infants born to
maternal users should not have withdrawal symptoms. However, 2
infants born to methamphetamine users did develop symptoms, as
did 4 whose heroin-using mothers claimed their last narcotic fix
was prior to 1 week before delivery. The author concludes that

the validity of these histories is doubtful and emphasizes a need
for careful evaluation of information derived from addicts. Likewise,
exact doses are rarely known and it is possible that addicts with
recent fixes whose infants were asymptomatic were on small doses.

Clues to aid diagnosis of neonatal addiction can be derived from a
history of maternal addiction, from maternal withdrawal symptoms,
or the presence of venereal disease, hepatitis, cellulitis, thrombophlebitis, septicemia, and illegitimacy, and the absence of prenatal
care. Diagnosis can be confirmed by demonstrating narcotic break-
down products in blood or urine if collected before the infant is
24 hours old. Sedative or narcotic therapy for the infant seems
unwarranted.

Ideally, the addict mother should have natural childbirth; any
sedatives or narcotics should be used sparingly. Newborns do not
have a psychic dependence on narcotics and should be permanently
cured once the umbilical is cut.

Neumann, Lois L. Drug abuse in pregnancy: Its effects on the fetus and newborn infant. In: Harms, Ernest, ed. <u>Drugs and Youth: The Challenge of Today</u>. New York: Pergamon Press, Inc., 1973. pp. 1-32. (164 references).

SUMMARY

Drug abuse among females in the childbearing age group is discussed, based on a review of the literature. There is ample clinical and chemical evidence that many drugs cross the placenta, including morphine and its derivatives and a number of the other drugs subject to abuse.

Drugs may exert two types of effects on the fetus--those which can be predicted on the basis of effects observed in adults, and those which are unique to the particular developmental stage of the fetus at the time of exposure. The former is exemplified by the neonatal narcotic withdrawal syndrome. Less is known about the effects of drugs of abuse on fetal development or the influence of different fetal developmental states on the actions of some of these drugs. It is important to document drug exposure during pregnancy as accurately as possible and to be alert to the possibility of abnormalities or alterations of physiology in infants of mothers with a history of such exposure. The medical problems related to drug abuse in pregnancy are compounded by the adverse social circumstances of the majority of habitual drug abusers in our culture, who live largely in urban areas with the highest rates of social pathology.

REVIEW OF THE LITERATURE

Effects Upon the Fetus and Newborn Infant

(1)   While addicts could be expected to be a high risk group, some authors noted a surprisingly low incidence of serious complications of pregnancy. One researcher found an increased frequency of toxemia and placental abnormalities as compared to the non-addict population delivered at the same hospital. An increased proportion of premature labors and breech deliveries was observed in all reported series. The frequency of breech presentation was probably secondary to the high proportion of low birth weight infants.

(2)   A treatment program during pregnancy increases the possibility of continued medical and social service supervision of mother and child after delivery. The occurrence of convulsions and sudden death at 1 to 2 months in several infants who had undergone methadone withdrawal is of special concern: intensive investigation is required to determine whether these serious reactions were caused by methadone, other drugs taken by the mothers, or some unrelated factor.

(3)   Various medical problems occur with increased frequency among addicts. The majority of these, including viral hepatitis, syphilis, tetanus, abscesses, septicemia, and bacterial endocarditis, are due to infections, some of which may secondarily affect infants born to addicted women.

(4)   The infant who has been chronically exposed to narcotics taken by his mother during pregnancy is suddenly cut off from the source of drugs at the time of delivery; abstinence symptoms may be expected to ensue.

There is general agreement that the cardinal symptoms are coarse tremors, hyperactivity, and irritability, and that a number of other symptoms frequently occur, including vomiting, poor feeding, greedy sucking, increased muscle tone, nasal stuffiness, sneezing, yawning, skin abrasions secondary to hyperactivity, persistent angry crying, sweating, and loose stools. Tachypnea, high fever, vascular collapse and convulsions have also been listed by some authors. Withdrawal symptoms usually begin during the first 24 hours of life. The infant whose mother has been drug-free for a week or more prior to delivery generally does not show signs of withdrawal. Symptoms of neonatal narcotic withdrawal have been reported as subsiding within a week or two and as persisting for as long as several weeks. It has been suggested by one study that heroin withdrawn infants have a relatively short period of acute symptomatology, which may be followed by a period of disturbed behavior manifested by sleeplessness and crying for 2 to 3 months, and hyperphagia, hyperacusis, and outbursts of screaming for as long as 6 months.

(5)   The narcotic withdrawal syndrome is a self-limited condition and, in milder cases, subsides in a few days with no specific therapy. A number of treatment regimens have been used for the management of infant narcotic withdrawal and most have been successful to some degree in controlling symptoms. Careful observation will determine which infants require no special treatment, which will respond to simple supportive measures, and which are in need of medication to control symptoms.

(6)   It is not known to what extent the addicted mothers' poor health and environmental circumstances, exposure to narcotic drugs, or some combination of factors, are responsible for the intrauterine growth retardation and premature delivery of their infants.

(7)   In the past, infants with narcotic withdrawal were given a poor prognosis for survival, with many fatalities attributed to dehydration or inanition. Recent experience indicates the neonatal mortality rate among these babies is not significantly higher than in other infants and that withdrawal symptoms, given appropriate management, cannot be considered an important cause of death. Further information on the long-term prognosis for infants born to addicts is badly needed.

16

(8)   Little has been established to date concerning the effects on infants of antenatal exposure to several of the commonly abused drugs. Until better information is available, clues as to the possible effects in infants born to mothers who have been taking amphetamines, barbiturates, hallucinogens, or tranquilizers must be sought in adult experience.

Gynecologic and Obstetric Considerations

(1)   Narcotic addicts frequently experience menstrual abnormalities. Amenorrhea is the most common, perhaps due to the physiological action of heroin or morphine. Regular menses return soon after withdrawal and while on methadone maintenance programs.

(2)   It is not known to what degree infertility is associated with addiction. The lack of menses does not necessarily imply lack of ovulation or fertility; one researcher reported a morphine addict who never menstruated after her third pregnancy but subsequently delivered 10 infants.

(3)   Using methods of substitution and gradual withdrawal, detoxification can be carried out at any stage of pregnancy except during labor.

Associated Medical Problems of Possible Significance to the Fetus

(1)   Hepatitis B antigen may be transmitted across the placenta but is rarely recoverable from the infant. There may be a link between antigenemia of mothers at delivery and premature births.

(2)   Syphilitic infection and the proteins responsible for biologic false positive reactions (BFP) can be transmitted to the fetus.

(3)   Tetanus during pregnancy would be a serious fetal threat even if the mother survived. Female addicts contract tetanus twice as often as males and should be immunized.

(4)   It is well established that intrauterine transmission of malaria may occur even in the absence of active disease symptoms in the mother. Some incidence of malaria is expected among pregnant addicts due to the return of servicemen from Vietnam with the disease.

(5)   Bacterial infections are usually acquired by the ascending route from the birth canal or by exposure during or following birth.

CONCLUSIONS

As abuse of multiple drugs becomes more widespread, more information is badly needed on not only the action of each individual drug but also on the effects of interactions between these drugs in various combinations on the infant in utero.

The pregnant addict of 75 years ago was likely to be a middle-class housewife without major complicating social pathology, who had become addicted unwittingly through the use of patent medicines with a high opium content. Surviving infants were probably cared for by the mother in a reasonably normal home environment. In contrast, the pregnant addict today is more often living a life characterized by inadequate food and housing, neglected health, prostitution, frequent arrests, and an unstable or non-existent family life. The greatest risks faced by the infant of the present-day addict are not those of acute neonatal withdrawal, but those related to the adverse conditions which accompany the mother's drug habit.

Neuberg, Roger. Drug dependence and pregnancy: A review of the
problems and their management. Journal of Obstetrics and
Gynaecology of the British Commonwealth, 77:1117-1122, December
1970. (32 references).

SUMMARY

Literature on drug-dependence during pregancy is summarized. Drug
dependence "on a periodic or continuous basis" included heroin, amphetamines, LSD, cannabis, and barbiturates.

Heroin produces a physical dependence in both mother and infant with
withdrawal management a life or death task in the case of the infant.
Amphetamine dependence is psychological, not physical and seems
to have no proven effect on infants. LSD is included because of its
"serious potential teratogenic effects." Cannabis is discussed because
it is the most widely abused drug and barbiturates because their use is
so widespread and "respectable" to the general public.

LITERATURE REVIEW

Heroin

Studies are cited showing that menstruation usually ceases after
months on heroin and returns shortly after withdrawal. A possible
explanation for this effect is that heroin and its metabolites cause a
neural block between the hypothalamus and pituitary gland and there
is therefore no stimulation of the secretion of gonadotrophin.

In a study comparing the case histories of 66 pregnant narcotic addicts
to all obstetric patients seen at the same hospital, medical complications and breech delivery were higher for addicted infants.

Many studies have reported a high incidence of prematurity, venereal
disease, and low birth weight among infants born to heroin-dependent
mothers. Methadone withdrawal was found to be possible (regardless
of the stage of pregnancy) in even the most heavily dependent narcotic
users within a few days.

When early signs of withdrawal are unrecognized and untreated, the
neonate may die. Symptoms include rapid respiration, grunting, rib
retraction, intermittent cyanosis, periods of apnoea, hyperactivity,
and trembling, twitching or convulsions, shrill high-pitched cry,
sucking of the fingers as if hungry, vomiting, diarrhea, hyperpyrexia,
excessive weight loss, sneezing cyanosis and incomplete mono reflex.

Management of infant narcotic withdrawal most often used methadone, paregoric elixir, phenobarbitone, and chlorpromazine.

Amphetamines

Four cases of methedrine dependence were analyzed. In terms of complications, it is possible that antepartum and postpartum haemorrhages were related to excessive methedrine dependence, but in general the drug had no adverse physical effects. Only one case was reported in which an infant showed drowsiness for four days possibly due to methedrine withdrawal.

LSD

Case studies show frequent abnormalities in fetuses of rats and mice given LSD during early pregnancies.

Chromosomal damage has not been conclusively proven in human leucocytes, but examples do exist of infants born with chromated breaks and malformations that could be related to LSD use by one or both parents.

Spontaneous abortion occurs more frequently among women who have taken LSD either before or during early pregnancy. There is a high incidence of abnormalities in the aborted fetuses; those reported included only cases where the father had taken the drug.

Cannabis

No chromosomal aberrations have been found in human leucocyte cultures given cannabis extract. The evidence is too scarce to draw conclusions.

Barbiturates

Although chronic barbiturate intoxification resembles chronic alcoholism and involves a danger of convulsions during withdrawal, there is no known risk to pregnancy caused by barbiturates taken in normal doses.

CONCLUSIONS

Heroin

There is such a lack of antenatal care among heroin addicted mothers that it is difficult to find which complications are due to heroin and which to physical deterioration, malnutrition, and ill health.

Amphetamines

It is possible that in the cases studied antepartum and postpartum hemorrhages were related to excessive methedrine use, but there is disagreement as to whether the drug has an effect on the cardio-vascular system. Since the drug produces a psychological de-pendence, not a physical one, it is likely to have no adverse physical effect in withdrawal either to mother or infant.

LSD

Spontaneous abortion occurs more frequently and there is a high in-cidence of abnormalities in the aborted fetuses among women who have taken LSD either before or during pregnancy.

The author feels that serious consideration should be given to ter-minating pregnancies in patients who have been on LSD because of the risk of fetal abnormality.

Desmond, Murdina M.; Schwanecke, Rebecca P.; Wilson, Geraldine S.; et al. Maternal barbiturate utilization and neonatal withdrawal symptomatology. The Journal of Pediatrics, 80(2):190-197, February, 1972.

DRUG	Heroin and Barbiturates		
SAMPLE SIZE	28		
SAMPLE TYPE	Parent-Child,	Treatment (inpatient) Treatment (outpatient)	
AGE	Infants		
SEX	Not Specified		
ETHNICITY	Not Specified		
GEOGRAPHICAL AREA	Houston, Texas		
METHODOLOGY	Longitudinal		
DATA COLLECTION INSTRUMENT	Medical Examination		
DATE(S) CONDUCTED	1962 to 1969		
NO. OF REFERENCES	26		

SUMMARY

Infants born to mothers taking barbiturates were compared to infants born to mothers addicted to heroin. The apparent barbiturate withdrawal syndrome differed from opiate withdrawal in the following ways: Infants with barbiturate exposure tended to be full-sized and had good 1 minute Apgar scores. This group also had onset of symptoms at a later age, and was less frequently jaundiced. The intensity and duration of behavioral changes was similar in both groups. Withdrawal symptoms in infants of epileptic mothers receiving barbiturates with other anticonvulsant drugs appeared to be milder and shorter than in infants of either

barbiturate or heroin addicts. All infants responded to a regimen
of frequent feeding, sedation, and diminished input of environmental stimuli.

METHODOLOGY

The stated purpose of this study was to outline the clinical characteristics of a possible neonatal withdrawal syndrome related to
maternal barbiturate use, and to compare the characteristics of
this syndrome with that encountered in infants of heroin addicts.

One sample group consisted of 15 infants born to mothers receiving barbiturates: 4 infants born to known barbiturate addicts
(throughout pregnancy), 4 infants of mothers receiving physician-
prescribed phenobarbital (last trimester of pregnancy), and 7
infants of epileptic mothers treated with phenobarbital in combination with other anticonvulsants, diphenylhydantoin or primidone
(last trimester).

The other sample was composed of 13 infants with congenital heroin addiction. Both groups of patients were seen over the same
period of time (1962 to 1969). The drug histories of the patients
were verified by reference to hospital records, and by interviews
with the mother, her family, and contacts. Mothers receiving
other or multiple psychoactive drugs were not included in this
report.

All patients were examined in the nurseries and nursery follow-up
clinic, and infants were entered into the study after detection during examination, or after referral by health centers. Examinations
were carried out monthly during the first 6 months of life and
thereafter at 3 month intervals.

FINDINGS

Of the 13 infants born to known heroin addicts, 5 weighed less
than 2,500 gm. at birth, although 4 were mature in appearance.
Birth depression (1 minute Apgar scores of 6 or less) occurred
in 6. Withdrawal symptoms (hyperactivity, disturbed sleep,
crying, and restlessness) occurred in all 13 infants, and there
were tremors in 12. The median age of onset of withdrawal
signs was 6 hours (range 10 minutes to 48 hours). Sedation was
given to 9 of the 13 infants for periods ranging from 3 to 67 days
(median, 18 days). Infants were discharged after signs of acute
withdrawal had subsided, when weight gain was adequate, and the
infant was able to sleep between feedings. When the infants returned
to the home setting, some symptoms recurred, most notably
sleeplessness and crying. These symptoms, along with constant
tremors when lying in a supine position and flexor extensor movements of the lower extremities, tended to diminish after 2 to 3

months. Hyperphagia, hyperacusis, and outbursts of screaming persisted in some through the first 6 months.

Barbiturate addicts: Four infants born to mothers with barbiturate addiction showed symptoms similar to those of the narcotic syndrome. All weighed over 2,500 gm. and had Apgar scores of 8 or better. Two of the infants exhibited in the nursery an onset of hyperexcitability, tremors, and restlessness at 63 hours, and 3 days, respectively. Two infants showed onset of symptoms at 4, and at 7 days, respectively. The duration of symptoms varied from 2 to 6 months. Sedation was required by 2 of the 3 babies seen as outpatients. The first improvement noted at home was the ability of the infant to sleep for several hours during the night.

Barbiturates as prescribed medication (90-120 mg. of phenobarbital daily): All infants were full term by weight and had good 1 minute Apgar scores. One of the four had evidence of "jitteriness" in the nursery at 30 minutes of age. Blood values for glucose and calcium were good. Because tremors and drying diminished by the second day, the infant was discharged on the 4th day. Tremors, quivering, constant hunger, sweating, hyperacusis, and very short sleep periods appeared on the 8th day and did not begin to improve until 5 weeks of age.

The other 3 showed no symptoms until a mean age of the 7th day, with peaks in intensity at 2 to 6 weeks. Feeding was frequently followed by gagging and vomiting.

Barbiturates as part of an anticonvulsant regimen (60 to 120 mg. of phenobarbital daily): One of the 7 babies was noted to have tremors, irritability, and a high-pitched cry, on the 2nd day. Glucose and calcium levels were physiologic. The infant required no sedation, improved during the 3rd and 4th days, and was discharged on the 5th day.

The other 6 neonates in this subgroup showed a median onset of symptoms at 7 days (range, 2 to 14 days). The intensity of symptoms appeared to be less in this group. The duration of symptoms had a median of 3 months (range, 2 to 4 months). There were minimal symptoms referable to the gastrointestinal tract. Anatomic variations and minor malformations in this group and in the others, and the regimen of management of all infants, were also discussed.

CONCLUSIONS

The functional immaturity of hepatic and renal systems in the newborn may explain the late onset of withdrawal symptoms in intrauterine barbiturate addiction. Care must be taken in comparing results of this study with other studies which were carried out within the first days of life, because the majority of the patients here demonstrated significant withdrawal signs only after discharge from the hospital. The late onset of neonatal symptoms of barbiturate withdrawal may preclude its detection in the hospital. The mother also may not be detected unless she shows clear signs of drug toxicity.

In both heroin and barbiturate neonatal withdrawal syndromes, the duration of symptoms is difficult to estimate because an acute phase may be followed by a subacute phase, lasting for months, and a marked influence of behavior is effected by the infants' environment (hospital nursery, home, parents, parent substitutes).

Bleyer, Werner A., and Marshall, Richard E. Barbiturate withdrawal syndrome in a passively addicted infant. <u>Journal of the American Medical Association,</u> 221(2): 185-186, July 10, 1972.

DRUG	Secobarbital (barbiturate)
SAMPLE SIZE	1
SAMPLE TYPE	Parent-Child
AGE	Infant
SEX	Male
ETHNICITY	White
GEOGRAPHICAL AREA	Seattle, Washington
METHODOLOGY	Case Study
DATA COLLECTION INSTRUMENT	Medical Examination
DATE(S) CONDUCTED	Not Specified
NO. OF REFERENCES	10

SUMMARY

This paper reported congenital barbiturate addiction in a child who sustained seizures and severe central nervous system hyper-irritability during the neonatal period, and again later in infancy. The authors hoped that increased awareness of the clinical manifestations and potential risks of congenital barbiturate addiction might lead to recognition and successful treatment of other cases of neonatal barbiturate withdrawal.

CASE STUDY

The subjects of this study were a white male infant and his mother, a 27-year-old primigravida. The mother, the wife of a physician and a registered nurse, had been addicted to barbiturates for as long as 5 years. Three days after delivery the mother sustained a grand mal seizure, and she later admitted haven taken secobarbital, 1.2 to 3.0 gm. daily during the pregnancy. Attempts at self-withdrawal led to generalized seizures on at least two occasions, and she had previously been hospitalized for secobarbital induced coma. Other barbiturates were also consumed, but abuse of alcohol, narcotics, cigarettes, and other drugs was denied.

The onset of labor began at 35 weeks gestation; uterine dystocia and intermittent fetal bradycardia on the day after admission necessitated cesarean section. Thiopental sodium administered following premedication did not provide adequate induction of anesthesia, and additional anesthesia with narcotic gases was required.

The child's Apgar scores were 7 and 9 at 1 and 5 minutes, respectively, and initially the infant appeared well. After admission to the nursery, however, the baby was found to be hyperactive, jittery, and tremulous. Some further clinical observations included: twitching of all extremities and clonic movements of the trunk, the Moro's and deep tendon reflexes were hyperactive, respirations were shallow, and oral feedings were regurgitated. Physical measurements, roentgenograms, various blood tests and cultures, and EKG were normal except for revealed bilateral perihilar and peribronchial infiltrates, which prompted treatment with a ten-day course of ampicillin and kanamycin.

The pulmonary infiltrates and respiratory distress cleared by the second day of life, but the hyperirritability increased so that there were present symmetrical clonic jerks, extreme jitteriness, incessant high-pitched screaming, frantic crying, and inability to suck.

Therapy with phenobarbital was initiated at 7 mg/kg of body weight/day. Phenobarbital therapy was reduced to 7, 5, and 3 mg/kg/day on the 5th, 7th and 9th days, respectively, and discontinued on the 11th day. The neonate's neurological distress subsided at the 10th day and the child was discharged in the care of the father on the 18th day of life.

One week later the mother left the hospital against medical advice and resumed taking secobarbital in dosages averaging 1.2 gm. daily. When the child had reached 4 months of age the mother was hospitalized for a suicide attempt with 7.0 to 10.0 gm of secobarbital. The next day the child developed vomiting, diarrhea, hypothermia, opisthonus, hyperreflexia, twitching of the extremities, and repetitive grand mal seizures. Intramuscular therapy with phenobarbital promptly controlled the seizures, but the other symptoms progressed in intensity. Again, a dosage of 6 mg/kg/day, intramuscularly, of phenobarbital eliminated the neurological distress by the 10th day. Thirteen days later the child was discharged, but was kept on a regimen of phenobarbital, 3/mg/kg/day.

It was later learned that the mother had given the child secobarbital for 2 to 3 months in daily doses averaging 60 mg, or approximately 13/mg/kg/day. It was noted that for sedation the generally recommended dosage is 2 to 3 mg/kg. The dosage of phenobarbital was gradually reduced and at the age of 2 years the child's EEG, growth and developmental parameters, and neurologic function were considered normal.

CONCLUSIONS

Although the authors' survey of the literature and two MEDLARS searches by the National Library of Medicine failed to produce any reports of neonatal barbiturate withdrawal, they feel strongly that their patient in this report exhibits such withdrawal symptoms. They include these points to substantiate their claims: evidence that the mother was physiologically dependent upon massive doses of short-acting barbiturates; demonstration of a high barbiturate tolerance during anesthesia, grand mal seizures and other signs of withdrawal 3 days post partum by the mother; absence of prenatal care, accessibility, etc.; and both illnesses in the infant developed abruptly on the day after termination of long-term barbiturate exposure, one being in utero.

Barbiturate withdrawal may be more likely to cause major motor seizures, and narcotic withdrawal may be more likely to exhibit autonomic and gastrointestinal distress. Both conditions are considered dangerous, but leave no apparent residual damage if recovery occurs. The slow improvement after phenobarbital therapy suggests to the authors that dosages in excess of 6 to 10 mg/kg/day may be required to adequately control barbiturate withdrawal symptoms in the infant.

II.   LSD

Long, Sally Y. Does LSD induce chromosomal damage and malformations? A review of the literature. Teratology, 6(1):75-90, 1972. (94 references).

SUMMARY

A review of 94 studies revealed no strong evidence either for chromosomal damage or teratogenicity as a result of LSD usage. Human subjects included abortuses, infants, children and adults of both sexes. The animal studies were conducted on rats, mice, kangaroo rats, rabbits, hamsters, and rhesus monkeys. Detailed tables of results from the 94 studies are included in the article.

Investigations for chromosomal damage were conducted in vitro and in vivo. The in vitro studies on humans utilized blood cells (lymphocytes); animal studies used hamster embryo cells and lung cells. The in vitro studies have demonstrated that a serum concentration of 0.01-10.0 ug/ml of LSD can cause human lymphocyte breakage in some cases while other investigators reported no increased breakage after the administration of 0.4-45.0 ug/ml (a hallucinogenic dose is 1.4 ug/kg body weight for humans which produces a serum concentration of 0.001 ug/ml).

The results of the in vivo studies are suspect due to the unknown and uncontrolled factors of LSD usage (number, dosage, and purity of past administrations) as well as types and quantities of other drugs taken concurrently, incidence of viral infections, and nutritional information. These studies included both former LSD users and subjects who were administered LSD in order to conduct controlled experiments. Even though an increase in chromosome breakage was found in 81% of 119 exposed subjects (in multiple studies), no correlation could be made between the number of breaks and the number of doses, total amount, nor time interval between last LSD dose and blood sampling. Results are complicated by the side variation in the frequency of chromosome breaks among subjects, as well as the wide range of mean chromosome breaks in the control groups (0.0 - 11.9%). In research on the same subjects before and after LSD use, no differences were found in the break frequencies for 42 patients (in two studies), while 3 out of 4 patients in another study showed a temporary increase in chromosome breaks, which returned to a normal level within 6 months.

In studies of the transmission of chromosome damage to offspring, either the meiotic cells of the adult LSD user himself or the children of parents who took LSD prior to or during pregnancy have been examined. Human male meiotic cells (testicular) showed no increased chromosomal breakage. (The author reported no studies on human female ovarian cells.) Seventeen out of 78 children (and one abortus) had increased breakage, with the greatest increases occurring in children whose parents took LSD during pregnancy. Breakage frequencies were also seen to parallel that in the mothers.

Of a reported 161 children of parents who took LSD prior to or during pregnancy, 7 had familiar defects and 16 had sporadic congenital disorders. The 5 cases of limb deficiencies among the 161 children could not be taken as evidence of the teratogenetic effect of LSD since there was no consistent pattern of malformations, no identifiable sensitive period during pregnancy, nor a critical dose level. Also, these deformities have a known frequency of occurrence in the population, and a bias could result from the more frequent reporting of malformed children whose parents took LSD than those who did not.

There does not appear to be well-documented evidence that LSD can cause chromosome breaks that may persist for lengthy periods of time, the risk for future generations seems small, and there is no strong evidence of teratogenic action of LSD in animals or man.

Titus, Robert J. Lysergic Acid Diethylamide: Its effects on human chromosomes and the human organism in utero. A review of current findings. The International Journal of the Addictions, 7(4): 701-714, 1972. (19 references).

SUMMARY

The findings of current studies in the area of LSD and chromosome damage are reviewed. The characteristic common to all studies was the conclusion that more experimentation is necessary before a definite answer can be obtained.

METHODOLOGY

The methodology typically used in LSD investigations is classified as in vitro or in vivo. The former involves human lymphocyte cultures exposed to LSD; the latter approach involves the actual intake, by an individual, of a known amount of LSD. Both approaches establish a relationship between the amount of chromosome damage and the concentration of LSD administered and the length of exposure.

The controls in these experiments would include a sample of blood not exposed to LSD compared to a sample from the same individual that was exposed, or a sample taken from a nonuser compared to one taken from a user.

FINDINGS: The Effect of LSD on Human Chromosomes

The earliest studies cited, by Smart and Bateman (1968), reported two in vitro studies showing a significant percentage of chromosomal abnormalities, and 7 in vivo studies which produced varying results. Smart and Bateman suggested that further studies would confirm that LSD affects human chromosomes adversely and possibly produces teratogenic effects on human offspring exposed in the fifth to sixth month of pregnancy. Smart and Bateman commented that more research should be done with germ cells rather than human lymphocytes when studying teratogenic effects in offspring.

Two in vitro studies (Kato and Jarvik, 1969; Corey, Andrews, McLeod, MacLean and Wilvy, 1970) showed a positive correlation between chromosomal damage and LSD. The percentage of chromosomal breaks (10.2% and 9.37% respectively) in their test samples was significantly higher than the breaks in their control samples (4.7% and 4.72% respectively).

Another study in 1969 (Judd, Brandkamp, and McGlothlin) compared a group of continuing users of LSD, a group which had discontinued its use, and a control group. Their percentage of chromosomal breaks was 0.32%, 1.8%, and 0.72% respectively. The fact that the control group had a greater percentage of breaks than the continuing users suggested that LSD had a negligible effect in this experiment.

Stenchever and Jarvis (1970) reported no significant difference in the breakage rates between their study and control groups. The percentage of breaks for each group ranged from 0-3.8%.

Other in vivo studies which found negligible differences between the LSD study group and control group include: (1) Corey, et al. (1970) whose ten nonusers showed a mean breakage of 5.7% before exposure and 4.9% after ingestion of LSD; (2) Tjio, Pahnke, and Kurland (1969) who attempted to relate size of dosage to number of breaks and observed no such relationship, nor any correlation between ingestion of LSD and increased chromosomal breaks; and (3) a study by Dorrance, Janiger, and Teplitz (1970) which showed that a control group had a greater percentage of breaks on the average than did a group of 14 subjects exposed to illicit LSD (0.79% to 0.76%).

The only in vivo study presented in this paper which showed a positive damage to the chromosomes of human lymphocytes was that of Nielsen and Tsuloi (1969). In two experiments, those exposed to LSD had chromosomal breaks of 4.3% and 2.5% as compared to 0.2% for the control group.

The most recent study available at the time of the author's writing was that of Gilmour, Bloon, Lele, Robbins, and Maximilian (1971), who compared drug users who had ingested LSD with drug users who had not ingested LSD. It was speculated that since there were chromosomal aberrations in a large number of subjects not using LSD, it is possible that such damage may be the result of other drugs, or a combination of drugs.

LSD and the Unborn

Three investigations done since 1968 are cited which show that exposure to LSD at various times in utero, will not necessarily cause chromosomal damage, abortion, or malformations. The first 2 investigations dealt only with women who had ingested LSD during pregnancy (results of these studies are presented in a statistical table). The third investigation concerned both a father and mother with a history of LSD ingestion before and during pregnancy. A normal son was born to them with no evidence of breaks or abnormal chromosomes.

33

There were five further clinical observations which showed that LSD, taken either during or before pregnancy, could very possibly be the cause of malformations. The first case involved a White mother whose child showed abnormalities heretofore only found congenitally among Puerto Ricans. The mother had used LSD at the time of conception. The baby died 40 days after birth.

A second case involved a child with a chromosomal aberration known as de novo D/D translocation with trisomy. Since neither parent was a carrier of this aberration, and both parents had taken LSD prior to conception only, it was suggested that LSD may have induced the abnormal chromosome arrangements in the germ cells of the mother. The child died shortly after birth.

The latter three cases were similar in that the offspring of the LSD ingesting parents exhibited limb abnormalities which were more severe on the right side, and in all three instances there was no evidence of chromosome damage in either mother or child.

The most extensive study regarding effects of LSD in utero conducted by McGlothlin, Sparkes, and Arnold (1970) included 148 pregnancies following parental intake of LSD with a median number of 25 exposures. The three major conclusions were:

1. There was no indication that abortions, premature births, or birth defects could be related to the use of LSD by the fathers before conception.

2. There was some indication that abortion, premature birth, and birth defects could be related to the ingestion of LSD by mothers before conception, but no clear-cut relationship could be established.

3. There was little evidence indicating a relationship between LSD and congenital defects.

CONCLUSIONS

The studies to date indicate that LSD causes negligible damage to the chromosomes of lymphocytes; however, there is evidence to support the hypothesis that LSD may have adverse effects on the normal development of humans in utero.

The effects of LSD on offspring would be of more consequence than its effects on adults, especially if the child's physical development is disturbed, or if the parent's germ cells are in some way damaged before conception by LSD.

Many drugs may cause irreparable damage to various parts of the body, without actually breaking chromosomes, by disturbing complicated enzymatic reactions. LSD is one of these drugs. This aspect of LSD could affect an adult, but more so a developing human embryo since chromosomes regulate the normal development of all body parts and systems. If LSD were to impair the function of chromosomes during this time, the result could be malformation.

Greenblatt, David J., and Shader, Richard I. Adverse effects of
LSD: A current perspective. <u>Connecticut Medicine</u>, 34(12):895-902,
December, 1970. (77 references).

<u>SUMMARY</u>

This article provided an overview of the dangers associated with
the use of LSD. Reports have implicated LSD in cytogenetic damage, in animals and man, with possible teratogenic or carcinogenic
results. Much of the research has been inconclusive and of poor
quality and has served to increase moral and legal resistance to
further research. Data has shown that cells cultured in media containing LSD have a significantly greater incidence of chromosomal
aberrations than cells from a control culture. Jarvik found that
a large number of chemical agents produce similar chromosome
damage <u>in vitro</u>. The clinical significance of this and the effects
<u>in vitro</u> were found to be uncertain. Sixteen studies examined the inci-
dence of chromosome abnormalities in users of LSD when compared
with that of controls who have not taken LSD. The term leukocyte
had been used loosely by most of the authors. This plus the poor
designs of the experiments combined to make the validity of the
findings questionable. The <u>in vitro</u> retrospective studies provided
very little useful knowledge as to the cytogenetic effect of LSD in
humans. Reports of the effect of LSD upon human pregnancy have
added very little useful information as to the possible role of LSD
as a teratogen. Studies were done by Berlin and Johnson and
McGlothlin; both surveyed pregnancies in which either mother or
father had taken LSD. The studies were poorly designed and the
significance of findings uncertain. McGlothlin did find an increase
in spontaneous abortions in LSD-taking mothers. Three cases were reported of infants with various congenital deformities of extremities
born to mothers who had ingested LSD and other drugs during the
first trimester of pregnancy. The authors felt that while such reports might be of interest, they did not establish a causal role of
LSD in the production of birth deformities. It was also noted that
these reports involved females from "high risk" populations.

There were 3 published studies in which the incidence of leukocyte chromosomal damage was determined in a single group of subjects both before and after a dose of LSD. Corey studied 10 patients who had received 200-600 mg. of LSD orally, and found no increase in chromosomal damage 24 hours after the single dose. The prospective studies were without the flaws found in the design of the retrospective studies; thus the results were found to be more meaningful. Additional findings were presented in an addendum to this paper, in which 2 or more cases were found of deformed infants born to mothers who used LSD during pregnancy. These and other findings did not alter the conclusions presented.

CONCLUSIONS

It has been suggested that LSD may cause chromosomal damage in animals and humans, with implications of a teratogenic or carcinogenic potential. At the present time the volume and quality of evidence were not found to be adequate to either confirm or rule out the possible adverse cytogenetic effect of LSD.

Smart, Reginald., and Bateman, Karen. The chromosomal
and teratogenic effects of Lysergic Acid Diethylamide: A review
of the current literature. Canadian Medical Association Journal,
99:805-810, October 26, 1968. (20 references)

SUMMARY

A review of existing research indicated uncertain results in terms
of chromosomal damage caused by LSD. There was some evidence
in one in vitro study, but very little evidence in the other, that the
extent of damage depends on dosage. Studies of the effects on the
chromosomes of human users produced mixed findings. The case
for chromosomal effects of LSD in human users has not been
proved. Further studies are warranted. Evidence for a teratogenic effect of LSD was found to be very strong but not unanimous
in animal studies.

REVIEW OF THE LITERATURE

Chromosomal Studies

Eight papers have examined the effects of various doses of LSD on
chromosomes. Six concluded that LSD did damage chromosomes,
2 concluded there was no effect.

Cohen, Marinello and Black carried out in vitro studies in which
leukocytes had been exposed to various concentrations of LSD.
Cells from 2 individuals were obtained and chromosomes were
examined after treatment with various amounts of LSD. The number of breaks in the LSD-treated group was double that of the
untreated; the rate of breakage ranged from 5-36.8%. Four hour
exposure produced the fewest overall number of breaks. Cohen,
Herschorn, and Frosch obtained similar findings with larger
samples.

Egozcue, Irwin, and Maruffo studied 50 LSD users and 14 nonuser
controls. LSD users had a mean breakage rate twice as high as
that of nonusers.

Cohen, Hirschorn, and Frosch found a high frequency of chromosomal abnormalities in LSD users. In addition, they examined the
chromosomes of 4 children born to 3 mothers who took LSD during
pregnancy. Two of the children whose mothers took LSD during
the third and fourth months had a high frequency of breaks;
2 exposed to low doses late in pregnancy showed 4.0 and 7.5% breaks.

Loughman, Sargent and Israelstam failed to find an effect of LSD on the chromosomes of users. Eight persons ingested LSD on 12 to 100 occasions; incidence of abnormalities was no higher than in 19 nonuser controls. Bender and Sankar failed to find LSD effects in 7 children.

According to Loughman, Sargent, and Israelstam, positive results may have occurred in certain studies where higher than usual doses of LSD were administered. Irwin and Egozcue have argued that Bender and Sankar failed to find chromosomal abnormalities in LSD takers because of the long interval between the last LSD dose and the examination of leukocytes, or because of the small number of chromosomes studied.

Teratogenic Effects

All studies reported were done on animals and are not abstracted here.

CONCLUSIONS

Chromosomal abnormalities found in LSD users could be incidental to their use of LSD, but related to the use of another drug.

Studies are needed where LSD is given before and at various stages during pregnancy. Studies are needed in which chromosome examinations are made of parents and offspring to determine the relationship between chromosomal and teratogenic effects. Evidence for LSD's harmful effects on chromosomes from small doses is insufficient. Three questions remain: the normal level of chromosome abnormalities, the minimal sample size needed for dependable analysis, and the contribution of other drugs to abnormalities.

Dumars, Kenneth W., Jr. Parental drug usage: Effects upon chromosomes of progeny. Pediatrics, 47(6): 1037-1041, June, 1971.

DRUG	LSD
SAMPLE SIZE	67
SAMPLE TYPE	Parent-Child
AGE	Infants (0-2)
SEX	Not Specified
ETHNICITY	Not Specified
GEOGRAPHICAL AREA	Irvine, California
METHODOLOGY	Controlled/Experimental
DATA COLLECTION INSTRUMENT	Laboratory/Examination
DATE(S) CONDUCTED	Not Specified
NO. OF REFERENCES	30

SUMMARY

Forty-seven infants born to users of LSD were examined clinically and the chromosomal karyotype was examined in 41. No evidence of increased chromosomal breakage or structural rearrangements could be found in those children born to the users of LSD, in comparison to the 20 controls under examination.

METHODOLOGY

The purpose of this report was to present the results of chromosomal studies performed upon infants relinquished for adoption,
whose parents had a history of LSD usage prior to and/or during
pregnancy. Patients came to the attention of the author when he
reviewed the records of all mothers and infants with either a medical or genetic problem, or a history of parental drug usage. The
parents had been referred to the Division of Adoptions in Orange
County, California, and all had been interviewed frequently in
various locations by a social worker.

A prepared form given to the parents of over 1,000 infants provided information concerning type, frequency, and timing of drug
usage. From this population a total of 47 cases of repeated LSD
usage could be documented. At least 30 of the mothers used LSD
prior to and during pregnancy, and at least one mother admitted to
250 "trips" during the 9 month pregnancy. Other drugs used
during this period by the parents included STP, cocaine, marijuana,
hashish, mescaline, barbiturates, amphetamines, tranquilizers,
antihistamines, and a few sniffed glue. Dosages were not documented because of reported inherent difficulties in such measures.

A leucocyte culture was obtained from the blood of 41 infants between birth and 3 months of age. Chromosomal karyotyping
figures were analyzed both visually and photographically. A control group consisted of 20 infants of parents of comparable age from
a group receiving routine well baby care by practicing pediatricians.
All control infants were well and had no history of illicit parental
drug usage.

FINDINGS

A total of over 3,000 figures were counted. Examination of karyo-
types in the experimental and the control group revealed that
chromosomal breakage occurred in less than 1.5%, and there was
no evidence of structural rearrangements in any cell. No significant statistical difference was found between the experimental and
the control groups. Eight infants exhibited clinical abnormalities
which the author will report at a later date.

CONCLUSIONS

The primary conclusion drawn was that the study was unable to
demonstrate increased chromosomal breakage or structural rearrangements in the chromosomal karyotype of infants born to
parents who were illicit users of LSD. Difficulties were mentioned
concerning evaluation of this study because information obtained

from the user concerning illicit usage cannot be considered highly accurate. However, the author feels strongly that a history of parental use of LSD is not a valid reason for failure of an agency to place, or a family to accept, a child of such parents relinquished for adoption.

Warren, R. J.; Rimoin, D. L.; and Sly, W. S. LSD exposure in utero.
Pediatrics, 45:466-469, March 1970.

DRUG	LSD
SAMPLE SIZE	5
SAMPLE TYPE	Parent-Child
AGE	Infants; Adults
SEX	Both Male and Female
ETHNICITY	Not Specified
GEOGRAPHICAL AREA	St. Louis, Missouri
METHODOLOGY	Case Study
DATA COLLECTION INSTRUMENT	Laboratory/Examination
DATE(S) CONDUCTED	1966-1967
NO. OF REFERENCES	14

SUMMARY

Because the teratogenic potential of LSD in humans is still uncertain,
the authors presented data on a clinically normal child with a normal
karyotype, who was repeatedly exposed to LSD during the first 4 months
of fetal life.

The mother reported that she conceived the infant on a day when both
she and her husband ingested LSD. She continued to ingest LSD during
the 2nd, 3rd, and 4th months of pregnancy, then discontinued LSD
ingestion throughout the pregnancy and lactation period.

Examination of the 8 month old child showed no abnormal chromosomal associations or significant number of breaks.

METHODOLOGY

The purpose of presenting this case report was to provide additional data on infants who have had in utero exposure to LSD, regardless of the presence or absence of congenital malformations, so that the teratogenic properties of the drug might be better evaluated.

The subjects of this report were a 37 year old father, a 36 year old mother, and their 8 month old son. While using LSD, peyote, and cannabis, the mother became pregnant. The mother's last menstrual period was on May 19, 1966, and she felt that she conceived on May 29, 1966, a day on which she ingested 320 μg and her husband 800 μg of LSD. Pure LSD was ingested by the mother again during the 2nd, 3rd, and 4th months of pregnancy. LSD ingestion was discontinued during the remainder of the pregnancy and the period of lactation. The mother continued to use cannabis regularly. She also ingested 3 buttons of peyote during the 4th month. The mother denies having ingested other drugs.

Leukocyte cultures were started on both parents and the 8 month old infant 5 weeks after the father ingested 800 μg and the mother ingested 320 μg of LSD. Control cultures were obtained with lymphocytes from a patient with Fanconi's anemia (positive control) and from one of the authors (negative control).

FINDINGS

The pregnancy was seen as otherwise uneventful and the child was born 2 weeks prior to the expected date of confinement. He weighed 6 lb., 8 oz. and was judged to be completely normal then and at 8 months of age. Dermatoglyphics were unremarkable.

Numerous breaks were found in the chromosomes of lymphocytes originating from the patient with Fanconi's anemia, but neither abnormal associations nor a significant number of breaks were found in the chromosomes of the parents, their child, or the author. Cells from the father did show, however, a large number of micronuclei scattered individually and sometimes in groups.

CONCLUSIONS

Since street LSD often contains other substances and LSD users tend to take other drugs as well as LSD, it is difficult to be certain whether observations by others of in vivo chromosomal damage are due to LSD, to the other drugs, or to a synergistic action requiring both. Because the infant son of this study was observed at 8 months of age, the authors cannot exclude the possibility that chromosomal damage would have been demonstrable earlier in life. This study does propose to demonstrate that intra-uterine exposure to pure LSD during the 2nd, 3rd, and 4th months, in addition to consistent exposure to cannabis, does not necessarily lead to abortion, persistent chromosome damage, or readily recognizable congenital malformations.

Stenchever, Morton A., and Jarvis, Jane A. Lysergic acid
diethylamide (LSD): Effect on human chromosomes in vivo.
American Journal of Obstetrics and Gynecology, 106(4):485-488,
February 15, 1970.

DRUG	LSD
SAMPLE SIZE	21
SAMPLE TYPE	Treatment (outpatient)
AGE	1 Infant, 20 Adults
SEX	Not Specified
ETHNICITY	Not Specified
GEOGRAPHICAL AREA	Cleveland, Ohio
METHODOLOGY	Controlled/Experimental
DATA COLLECTION INSTRUMENT	Laboratory/Examination
DATE(S) CONDUCTED	Not Specified
NO. OF REFERENCES	8

SUMMARY

Chromosome analysis was carried out on the blood lymphocytes
of 12 adults who used LSD and one infant born to an LSD user, and
this was compared with 8 control subjects. No significant difference in chromosome gaps, breakage, or abnormal forms was
found between groups. Possible reasons for differences in results
between in vivo studies, and between in vivo and in vitro studies
were given.

METHODOLOGY

The present study was performed with 13 persons, 12 of whom had ingested LSD as adults, and one patient, a 1 1/2 year old child, who had been exposed to the drug as a fetus. A control group, consisting of 8 adults ranging in age from 17 to 45, was selected from a pool of patients and resident physicians, none of whom presented a history of recent exposure to agents which are known to cause chromosome breakage.

Test procedures involved taking a 10 cc. sample of venous heparinized blood from each adult subject and exposing it to phytohemagglutinin for 30 minutes. After being centrifuged at 500 r.p.m., the supernatent plasma containing leukocytes was then added to flasks containing Medium TC 199 (GIBCO) with penicillin and streptomycin added. Cultures were incubated for 72 hours at 37° C, and 90 minutes prior to harvesting, 0.2 ml. of 1×10^{-6} M colchicine was added to each flask. Slides were stained with carbolfuchsin and coded for blind scoring.

Scoring involved checking representative slides from each culture for gaps, chromatid breaks, isochromatid breaks, and abnormal forms, such as rings, dicentrics, quadriradials, and triradials.

FINDINGS

No significant differences were noted for gap or break rates between the study group and the controls. Only 2 LSD patients had apparent increases in gap rates, but no significant breakage was seen in either case. No abnormal forms were seen in any of the patients studied but one quadriradial form was seen in one of the control cultures.

CONCLUSIONS

The authors detailed some of the possible reasons for demonstrations of in vivo chromosome breakage in some studies and not in others. Procedural differences between laboratories was held to account for at least some of these differences, because those reporting higher breakage rates tend to use less complete media for culturing cells. Therefore, these groups also report higher breakage rates in their controls as well. Samples drawn from capillary blood as opposed to venous blood was seen as another source of discrepancies.

Another problem involves estimation of dose levels taken by patients because of the rather crude form of the drug used in most cases. A large variation in blood levels of the drug achieved in the various cases within the study group must therefore be expected. The authors feel that it is therefore probable that the total reported dose cannot be accurately correlated with the development of breaks. Also, controls for the influence of other agents either individually or in concert with LSD cannot be overlooked.

Possible pitfalls in attempts to compare in vivo and in vitro data were also outlined. For example, body regulatory mechanisms may protect cells that would not be protected in vitro. Also, natural forces of selection may tend to favor the unaffected cells in vivo more than in vitro when there are cells damaged. Further, the times required for a complete cell cycle of lymphocytes are different between in vitro and in vivo conditions, and it is likely that lymphocytes are more susceptible to LSD at certain times in the cell cycle than at other times. Therefore, the authors would expect that proportionately fewer cells in vivo are at risk at any given time than would be the case in vitro because of the difference in cycle time.

Hirschborn, Kurt, and Cohen, Maimon M. Drug-induced chromosomal aberrations. Annals of the New York Academy of Sciences,
151(2):977-897, 1968.

DRUG	LSD and Mitomycin (antibiotic)
SAMPLE SIZE	Not Specified
SAMPLE TYPE	Not Specified
AGE	Cross-Age
SEX	Both Male and Female
ETHNICITY	Not Specified
GEOGRAPHICAL AREA	Not Specified
METHODOLOGY	Controlled/Experimental
DATA COLLECTION INSTRUMENT	Laboratory/Examination, Experimental Test
DATE(S) CONDUCTED	Not Specified
NO. OF REFERENCES	41

SUMMARY

A variety of effects of pharmacological agents on chromosomes in
vitro were discussed. LSD was shown in a number of tests to be
capable of producing chromosomal aberrations. Some of these
effects appear to have occurred in vivo in human material. It was
postulated that such chromosomal damage could be produced by a
variety of mechanisms, and could result in an increased incidence
of neoplasia in the exposed individual, in addition to abortions or
possible chromosomal rearrangements in future generations resulting in fetal wastage and damage.

METHODOLOGY

This study directed its attention to the procedures used to assay the activity of compounds of pharmacologic interest relevant to their effect on chromosomes, and the possible significance of this effect.

The test employed was phytohemagglutinin-stimulated peripheral lymphocytes which are incubated for a 72-hour period in commercially available "microculture kits." Fibroblastic cell cultures derived from various tissues can also be used. The test compound was added to these cultures at various concentrations and for different lengths of exposure. Response curves were then formulated with respect to both time and dose.

One parameter of the tests mentioned was the effect of the drug on cell division, i.e., mitotic rate indices. Closer attention was paid, however, to methods of scoring possible chromosomal aberrations. Four major abnormalities were described. They included chromatid breaks, isochromatid breaks, dicentrics, and translocations. Also, 4 different classes of genetic consequences of these aberrant exchanges were described.

FINDINGS

1.   In the first study lymphocytes from 6 normal subjects were stimulated to divide by the addition of phytohemagglutinin. LSD was added to the test cultures in concentrations ranging from 0.001 to 10 ug/ml from 4 to 48 hours prior to harvest of the cells. Cultures from the same subjects without LSD served as controls. One-hundred cells per treatment per subject were examined in a double-blind procedure. All doses and all periods of exposure produced an increase in abnormalities which ranged to over 4 times the control values of 3.9% of abnormal cells. Some types of exchanges and breaks were not found in the control.

2.   This study used 18 patients ingesting LSD, and 12 age-matched controls, with their lymphocytes cultured in the presence of phytohemagglutinin. About 100 metaphases were scored, again on a double-blind basis. The "dry-free" controls showed a range of break frequencies of 2.0 - 5.5%, with a mean of 3.8% based on the scoring of 2,674 metaphases. The 18 adults with LSD ingestion histories demonstrated a break frequency of from 5.3 - 25.1%, with a mean of 13.2% based on 4,282 metaphases scored. There was consistency among results from the same individual, different culture tubes, and different culture times. There was no apparent correlation between the rate of LSD use or dose, and breakage rate, nor was there any correlation in this group with any combination of drugs, to the exclusion of LSD and breakage rates.

3.   The chromosomes of 4 children exposed to LSD in utero were examined. Two of the children whose mothers had taken doses of 300 to 600 ug/dose showed highly elevated break frequencies. Two children born to a mother who took only 50 to 100 ug/dose showed only a very mild elevation in breaks. A child whose mother had taken large doses of LSD and who was exposed to no other drugs during pregnancy, and had not been exposed to LSD since birth, still showed 13% breaks 2 1/2 years after birth.

4.   Exposure to chlorpromazine on the day of bleeding was associated with high rates of chromosome breakage.

5.   One patient taking diphenylhydramine up to the day of testing showed a mild increase in chromosome breakage.

CONCLUSIONS

The authors speculate that chlorpromazine exerts only a transient effect, but that the effects of LSD are long lasting. They conclude that there are no answers at this time to the question of risk associated with drug ingestion, as it affects the health of an individual and/or his progeny. Mention is made of some autosomal recessive diseases which exhibit in cells of neoplastic origin chromosomal aberrations not unlike those seen after LSD or mitomycin exposure. The authors see exposure to chromosome-breaking agents as a possible future source of increased incidence of leukemia and other neoplasms.

Because of transplacental transport of LSD and subsequent chromosome damage in the exposed fetuses, the authors fear possible congenital defects and abortions may result. In their own studies the authors saw no direct correlation between behavioral disorders, dosage, frequency, time since last dose, and the incidence of chromosomal damage in the group studied, nor were there any obvious physical or behavioral abnormalities noted in the 4 children exposed in utero. However, since the potential for great danger in the use of such agents lies in potential chromosome damage to the gametes, and the carrier of such damaged gametes may be clinically normal, the authors expressed the fear that the consequences of the damage may not appear for several generations.

Jacobson, Cecil B., and Berlin, Cheston M. Possible reproductive detriment in LSD users. <u>Journal of the American Medical Asssociation,</u> 222(11):1367-1373, December 11, 1972.

DRUG	Hallucinogens, Multi-Drug
SAMPLE SIZE	148 Pregnancies (140 mothers)
SAMPLE TYPE	Volunteer
AGE	65 Fetal, 83 Infants
SEX	Both Male and Female
ETHNICITY	White
GEOGRAPHICAL AREA	Washington, D.C. area
METHODOLOGY	Case Studies
DATA COLLECTION INSTRUMENT	Interviews, Laboratory/Examination
DATE(S) CONDUCTED	1968 to 1970
NO. OF REFERENCES	16

SUMMARY

One-hundred and forty pregnant women and their consorts with personal histories of LSD usage (either in both parents or only one parent) were followed through 148 pregnancies. There were 83 live newborns; 8 had major congenital defects. There were 65 abortions; 53 therapeutic and 12 spontaneous. Four of 14 embryos from therapeutic abortions showed gross anomalies. Forty-three percent of first-trimester pregnancies ended in spontaneous abortions. Four of 8 serial pregnancies resulted in defective embryos or infants. Eight of 12 women have been unable to conceive again over an 18 month period.

The ingestion of other illicit drugs, the presence of infectious disease, and marginal maternal nutrition precluded a definitive correlation of increased reproductive risk with LSD ingestion.

METHODOLOGY

Personal interviews were conducted to assess each mother's history of exposure to other drugs, venereal disease, infectious disease during pregnancy, and prenatal nutrition (all available consorts were also interviewed). The patients were characterized as white, middle- to upper-middle-class Americans, approximately one-half of whom had adopted a "hippie" lifestyle (the other half were in sympathy with hippie lifestyles but lived more conventional lives).

The authors examined the newborn infants whenever possible, with follow-up examinations at 2 weeks, 6 weeks, 3 months, 6 months, and then at 6 month intervals, with the longest follow-up being 2 1/2 years at the publication of the article. Fetal tissue from 14 abortuses was also examined.

Five LSD samples given to the authors by the patients for analysis varied in strength from 50 ug to 125 ug. The number of doses taken by the mothers of the eight abnormal infants varied from zero to 400 prior to conception.

FINDINGS

Ten of the pregnancies occurred with paternal LSD use only, with 7 live births, 3 abortions, and no abnormal infants in this group. Of the two infants that died of gross abnormalities shortly after birth, neither mother took LSD at any time during her pregnancy. All of the patients reported marijuana use, and 82% had used amphetamines. Other drugs taken by the patients included peyote, mescaline, dimethyltryptamine, narcotics (6 heroin addicts out of 26 users), STP, and barbiturates. Possible mutagens ingested included coffee, tea, cyclamates, and tobacco. Thirty-six percent of these mothers experienced x-ray exposure during pregnancy.

Of the 65 abortions, 53 were therapeutic (performed for psychiatric indications). Fourteen of these abortuses were intact enough for examination; four of the 14 showed prominent midline fusion defects. Of the 7 spontaneous abortions, 4 were abnormal embryos with neural-tube fusion defects. Previous studies indicate an overall abnormality rate of 43% for spontaneous abortions (compared to the 57% in the small sample examined in this study). The peak frequency for abnormalities in electively terminated pregnancies has been found to be 4% (in a study involving 1,213 embryos), while 29% (4 out of 14) were found to be abnormal in this study.

CONCLUSIONS

The authors compared the incidence of major congenital anomalies in this population (8 of 83 live-born infants) with the incidence in a home for unwed mothers where pregnancy outcomes have been monitored since 1962. That rate has remained stable at 6 per 1,000 live births. Based on this data, the incidence of major congenital anomalies in the offspring of a group of drug users was from 10 to 20 times that expected for the American population. The multiple factors possibly responsible for fetal defects in this group of women (prenatal nutrition, viral infections, heavy use of other drugs, etc.) preclude the implications of LSD use as the definitive teratogenetic agent in these case histories.

Eller, J. L. , and Morton, J. M. Bizarre deformities in offspring of user of lysergic acid diethylamide. New England Journal of Medicine, 283:395-397, August 20, 1970.

DRUG	Hallucinogens
SAMPLE SIZE	1
SAMPLE TYPE	Parent-Child
AGE	Neonate
SEX	Female
ETHNICITY	White
GEOGRAPHICAL AREA	Denver, Colorado
METHODOLOGY	Case Study
DATA COLLECTION INSTRUMENT	Medical Exam
DATE(S) CONDUCTED	Not Specified
NO. OF REFERENCES	8

SUMMARY

An infant with a rare combination of severe congenital deformities was born to a woman with a history of using lysergic acid diethylamide. Previously described patients bearing a similarity to this infant were of Puerto Rican parents, most of consanguineous marriage, and in none of these cases was use of this drug indicated. The current state of knowledge of the effects of the compound is such that no definite inference can be made about the current case. All reported cases similar to this one appear to have been due to an unusual recessive mode of inheritance or chromosomal aberration.

METHODOLOGY

The subject of this case report, a female neonate, was the first child of unrelated parents, both native-born citizens of the United States. The medical history of the father was unknown. The 19-year-old mother had no past history of serious illness and no prior exposure to ionizing radiation except routine chest roentgenograms.

The mother was a cigarette smoker who admitted using LSD on a single occasion at about the time of conception. An estrogen preparation was also taken early in the first trimester to induce menstruation, which was unsuccessful. First trimester bleeding was treated conservatively with medroxyprogesterone acetate. No other illnesses, problems, or drug usage were known to the authors during pregnancy, the mother's first. A thorough medical examination was performed, including roentgenograms and an autopsy. Photographs and roentgenograms of the child are shown.

FINDINGS

The infant, a breech delivery who failed to breathe spontaneously, responded immediately to intubation. There were many deformities present at birth: short neck, left hemithorax smaller than the right, protuberant abdomen, thoracolumbar rachischisis, club feet, longer than normal fingers.

Roentgenograms revealed the following: multiple hemivertebras, neural-arch defects, severe thoracolumbar lordosis, and craniolacunia.

At the age of 6 days an anuric condition had been present for 40 hours. A bladder tap yielded normal urine. A cystogram demonstrated a persistent urachus and a rectovesical fistula. The bladder was large and trabeculated. Contrast material in the colon passed from the bladder through the fistula.

At age 40 days labored respirations and cyanosis developed. Autopsy confirmed the internal abnormalities mentioned above. Other findings include: horseshoe kidney, single midline adrenal gland, Arnold-Chiari malformation, with hydrocephalus fusion of the frontal lobes of the brain and a bilateral interstitial pneumonia. Chromosome studies gave normal results.

CONCLUSIONS

The authors related this single case to some reported infants who showed remarkably similar clinical and roentgenographic features, especially those of the chest and spine. The authors postulate an autosomal recessive mode of inheritance for at least some of these latter cases. These infants were all born of Puerto Rican parents, with no history of LSD use.

The importance of the observation of deformities like this in white parents is held to be unknown. The authors mention some other cases where mild deformities have been associated with LSD use. However, they point out that more knowledge is needed before LSD use can be strongly related to the deformities in their patient, especially since normal results were obtained from chromosomal studies.

III.　　HEROIN

Barton, William I. A statistical study of infants born with withdrawal
symptoms in the District of Columbia. Medical Annals of the
District of Columbia, 42(6):287-290, June 1973.

DRUG	Heroin
SAMPLE SIZE	7 hospitals
SAMPLE TYPE	Parent-Child; Treatment (inpatient)
AGE	Infants
SEX	Not Specified
ETHNICITY	Not Specified
GEOGRAPHICAL AREA	Washington, D. C.
METHODOLOGY	Statistical Study
DATA COLLECTION INSTRUMENT	Questionnaires
DATE(S) CONDUCTED	1972
NO. OF REFERENCES	2

SUMMARY

Drug usage (particularly heroin usage) by expectant mothers can
result in infants born with the withdrawal syndrome. Most of the
research to date on the effect of drugs on the fetus and on the newborn infant has been qualitative, of general scope, or based on
experience within a specific institutional setting. In order to obtain
quantitative information on the problem of infants born with withdrawal symptoms, permitting statistical analyses of trends, a survey
was conducted in 1972 of 9 hospitals within the District of Columbia.
Of the 9 hospitals contacted, some information was received from
7 for a response rate of 78 percent. This statistical study is based
on the information supplied.

METHODOLOGY

The survey instrument was a letter addressed by name to the Chief of the Department of Pediatrics for each of the 9 hospitals. Information requested included:

(1) The number of infants born with withdrawal symptoms and the total number of infants born, by month, for the first 4 months of 1972;

(2) Whether it would be possible to obtain the same information for 1971;

(3) Whether the information supplied could be subdivided according to race and residence of mother;

(4) Whether the hospital had a screening process in which mothers were queried prior to delivery about possible drug use and, if so, what proportion of the mothers who delivered in the hospital were queried; and

(5) Of the mothers queried, what proportion received a query during a prenatal visit rather than at the time of delivery.

Provision was made in the survey for follow-up letters and telephone calls when necessary.

FINDINGS

Information supplied in response to the query was quite variable. No hospital had on hand or ultimately supplied all of the information requested. For 1971, the 4 hospitals which provided data on the number of infants born with withdrawal symptoms accounted for approximately 13,591 of the 25,024 births occurring at the 9 hospitals included in the survey (for about 54 percent of these births). The overall rate for 1971 for these hospitals (4.0 infants with withdrawal symptoms per 1,000 births) was lower than the rate which occurred for the first 4 months of that year (4.1 infants with withdrawal symptoms per 1,000 births).

For the first 4 months of 1972, the same 4 hospitals accounted for about 3,917 births out of some 7,225 births occurring at the hospitals included in the survey (or about 54 percent of these births). The rate (5.4 infants born with withdrawal symptoms per 1,000 births) was only slightly higher than that shown for these hospitals in 1971 during an identical time period. Among the 7 hospitals in the survey which provided data for the first 4 months of 1972, there were 32 infants with withdrawal symptoms out of some 6,257 births, resulting in a rate of 5.1 infants with withdrawal symptoms per 1,000 births.

The majority of infants with withdrawal symptoms were born in the District of Columbia General Hospital. For 1971 this hospital had a rate of 10.9 infants born with withdrawal symptoms per 1,000 births, with quite a variation in monthly rate. For the first 4 months of 1972 there were 10 infants with withdrawal symptoms out of some 1,106 births, resulting in a somewhat lower rate (9.0 infants with withdrawal symptoms per 1,000 births).

The hospitals provided race and residential data only for infants born with withdrawal symptoms. Thus it was not possible to construct any other rates. Only 5 hospitals provided information as to whether there was a screening process in which mothers were queried prior to delivery about possible drug use. Three of these hospitals responded that there was no uniform screening process.

CONCLUSIONS

There are a number of limitations to obtaining reliable and valid data on the number of infants born with withdrawal symptoms within a geographical boundary. These limitations include nonspecific symptoms which may not be recognized as drug withdrawal, inadequate staffing of medical records departments, incomplete records on infants born with withdrawal symptoms and data retrieval systems that are outmoded and do not lend themselves to statistical analyses. In addition, there seems to be a serious error of omission in the prenatal programs conducted by some hospitals in the District of Columbia. Data provided allows no statement on the proportion of mothers delivering in the surveyed hospitals who are queried about drug use prior to actual delivery or, for those mothers who are queried, on the proportion queried at the time of a prenatal visit as opposed to just prior to delivery. It would seem that a query directed to all expectant mothers about drug usage would result in a lessening of morbidity and mortality connected with drug withdrawal occurring at the time of childbirth.

Lin-Fu, Jane. <u>Neonatal Narcotic Addiction</u>. (Children's Bureau, Welfare Administration, U.S. Department of Health, Education, and Welfare.) Washington, D.C.: U.S. Government Printing Office, 1967. 11 pp. (16 references).

SUMMARY

This article presented an overview of the research that has been done on the health problems of addicted pregnant women and the problems of infants with neonatal narcotic addiction. Not only are the women high-risk obstetrical patients, but most of their babies are born addicted and suffer a high neonatal mortality and morbidity rate.

FINDINGS

Incidence

Although the incidence of narcotic addiction in pregnant women is often difficult to determine, 300 infants in New York in 1965 were diagnosed as suffering from neonatal narcotic addiction. Perhaps 400-500 infants were born to addicts in New York in 1966. Federal Bureau of Narcotics statistics, as of December 31, 1965, reported 57,199 active narcotic addicts in the United States. Of these about 18% were females. Smith, et al., reported that in 1965, 77% of a sample of patients seen at the Lexington, Kentucky hospital were 25 or younger. Most female narcotic addicts, then, would have a long potential reproductive period. Therefore narcotic addiction in pregnant women cannot be a rare occurrence in this country.

Health Problems of the Mother

Lack of prenatal care seemed common among addicts. Among 66 addicted pregnant women, Stein found that the average number of prenatal visits was less than 1 per patient. High incidence of obstetrical complications was found among addicted women. Rosenthal found in the histories of 16 patients, 35 abortions and 6 still births. Stern found toxemia of pregnancy in 15.1% of 66 patients, 12% breech-presentation, and abruptio placenta in 9%. Premature labor was also cited as a frequent complication of pregnancy in addicts. A high incidence of postpartum complications was also noted. Stern found that 8 out of 40 pregnant addicted women had a positive serology. Among other complications often seen were malnutrition, serum hepatitis, and venous thrombosis. Twenty percent of Stern's sample of 66 addicted women signed out of the hospital against advice after delivery. Lack of adequate postpartum care among those women was felt to be a cause for concern, particularly because of the high incidence of complications.

Neonatal Narcotic Addiction

Most, but not all, infants born to addicted mothers developed narcotic withdrawal syndrome. It was estimated that 83 to 91% of infants of addicted mothers were born addicted. If more than a week had passed between the mother's last narcotic dose and delivery, the infants were usually symptom free.

The first clue to neonatal withdrawal symptoms may be violent fetal kicking. Respiratory distress may occur at birth. Often these infants appeared normal at birth, but about 80% became symptomatic within the first 24 hours. Central nevous system hyperirritability was the most frequent manifestation of narcotic withdrawal in new-born infants. This was characterized by restlessness, protracted cry of a shrill and piercing quality, jumpiness, etc. Diarrhea and vomiting were common. Severity of symptoms appeared to be correlated with the dosage of the drug taken by the mother and possibly to the route of administration. Goodfriend, et al., found the overall mortality rate among addicted new-born infants was 34%, and 93% among untreated symptomatic infants. Mortality among symptomatic infants who received no treatment was generally reported to be high. High incidence of low birth weight was found. Stern reported that 18.5% of infants in his series were premature. Others reported similar findings. Increased susceptibility to infection was enhanced by debilitation, skin excoriation, and prolonged hospitalization.

CONCLUSIONS

Health workers must depend on evidence other than a positive history of addiction or withdrawal symptoms in the mother when substantiating a diagnosis of neonatal narcotic addiction. The worker must look for signs in the mother's history such as hepatitis or thrombophlebitis. Needle marks, miosis, tatoos and other signs of addiction might present further clues.

It is generally agreed that narcotic withdrawal should not be attempted late in pregnancy, but no optimum time in pregnancy has been established.

Treatment of infants should not start before onset of withdrawal symptoms. A number of medications have been used along with supportive therapy. Between a few days and a few weeks, gradual withdrawal of the medicine may be attempted.

Long-term care of these infants following drug withdrawal remains a problem, and is dependent upon the successful treatment and rehabilitation of the addicted mother.

Krause, Samuel O.; et al. Heroin addiction among pregnant women and their newborn babies. American Journal of Obstetrics and Gynecology, 75(4):754-758, April 1958.

DRUG	Heroin
SAMPLE SIZE	18
SAMPLE TYPE	Treatment (inpatient)
AGE	Neonates
SEX	Both Male and Female
ETHNICITY	Not Specified
GEOGRAPHICAL AREA	New York City
METHODOLOGY	Case Studies
DATA COLLECTION INSTRUMENT	Observations
DATE(S) CONDUCTED	1955
NO. OF REFERENCES	2

SUMMARY

Eighteen pregnant heroin addicts and their newborn babies were studied. The cases were analyzed as to method of delivery, postpartum treatment and complications, fetal salvage and fetal deaths, birth weight, fetal complications and treatment. Four of the 18 infants died, 5 were treated successfully with methadone and the others survived withdrawal under supervision of the obstetric department.

FINDINGS

Only 4 patients had prenatal care, and 11 cases of antepartum complications were observed. All responded to treatment. Premature labor was experienced by 39 percent. Most patients had received an injection just prior to admission and did not experience withdrawal symptoms until 6 to 24 hours later.

Sixteen mothers experienced postpartum withdrawal in varying degrees. All left the hospital within 5 days although they had been offered methadone and were encouraged to stay until they were drug-free. One case of postpartum psychosis received psychiatric care.

Only one baby weighed more than 6 1/2 lbs. The average weight was 5 lbs. 13 ozs. Five weighed less than 5 1/2 lbs.

Fifteen neonates developed withdrawal symptoms within 1 to 56 hours after birth. Characteristic syndromes included: excess greenish or brownish mucus which interfered with breathing; abnormal tremor of limbs within 6 to 18 hours; vomiting; inability to nurse; difficulty swallowing; respiratory crisis; irritability and crying spells.

The four neonate deaths occurred on the 6th, 7th, 8th, and 18th day of life. All were born to mothers with antepartum complications; one mother had undergone withdrawal one day prior to delivery. All 4 neonates experienced withdrawal symptoms.

Autopsy showed: (1) subdural hemorrhage; (2) subtentorial hematoma; (3) atelectasis; (4) polycystic kidneys; (5) severe tolipes equinovarus; and (5) Mongolism.

The surviving babies were usually asymptomatic within 6 to 7 days.

CONCLUSIONS

It was not possible to correlate the severity of neonatal withdrawal with the mother's degree of withdrawal because there were no controls on the mother's supply of heroin from outside the hospital.

At the time of this study the pediatric department began using methadone to manage infant withdrawal with apparent success. Barbiturates, belladonna, paregoric and special formulas appeared to have no value in the management of the neonates.

Stone, Martin L., et al. Narcotic addiction in pregnancy.
American Journal of Obstetrics and Gynecology, 109(5): 716-723,
March 1, 1971. (10 references).

DRUG	Opiates
SAMPLE SIZE	382
SAMPLE TYPE	Treatment (inpatient)
AGE	Infants, Adolescents, Adults (Average age 26.7)
SEX	Female Addicts Both Male and Female Infants
ETHNICITY	61% Black, 23% Puerto Rican, 16% White
GEOGRAPHICAL AREA	New York City
METHODOLOGY	Exploratory/Descriptive
DATA COLLECTION INSTRUMENT	Observations, and Laboratory/Examination
DATE(S) CONDUCTED	1960 to 1969
NO. OF REFERENCES	10

SUMMARY

A study of 382 pregnant addicts in New York City reflected significant problems: over 90% had inadequate prenatal care; the
incidence of complications (prematurity, toxemia, breech birth
and precipitate labor) was higher than in the general clinic population. Prostitution increased the incidence of venereal disease
and hepatitis. Over 70% of the infants manifested congenital neonatal addiction with clinically recognizable withdrawal symptoms.
Hyperactivity of the autonomic nervous system was evidenced by
diaphoresis, diarrhea, and rhinorrhea. Hypertonicity and shrill

crying were frequent. Infants were premature by date, and 50% manifested retarded intrauterine growth. The severity of the symptoms was related to the maternal dose.

METHODOLOGY

Observations were made of 382 pregnant addicts delivered of infants between 1960 and 1969 at Metropolitan Hospital in East Harlem.

FINDINGS

Addicts

The ratio of addicts to total deliveries increased from 1:164 in 1960 to 1:47 in 1969. Average age was 26.7; there was an increase in teenage patients from 2 in 1960 to 26 in 1969. Racially, 61% were Negro, 23% Puerto Rican, and 16% White. Approximately one-third were married. Parity reflected age; fertility did not seem to be adversely affected. All used heroin; 20% also used barbiturates and tranquilizers. Duration of addiction ranged to over 20 years. More than 80% evidenced drug use on the day of admission in labor.

Obstetric complications included premature labor, breech presentation, premature rupture of membranes and toxemia. Medical complications were anemia, syphilis, and infectious hepatitis. All may be explained on the basis of inadequate prenatal care. There were few serious complications. Breech presentation may reflect the increased prematurity rate with many low birth weight infants. The many positive serologies were related to the fact that prostitution is common as a way to support the drug habit. Average length of labor was short. It has been suggested that patients off heroin have increased uterine irritability. After delivery, withdrawal symptoms were manifested in nausea, tremors, sweats, abdominal pain, cramps, and yawning.

Neonates

Almost half of the infants were premature by weight; 40.5% were 38 weeks gestation or over. Neonatal addiction and withdrawal symptoms occurred among 67.4%. Onset of symptoms ranged from birth to 4 days. Onset and frequency depended on the amount of heroin taken by the mother. Central nervous system irritability was the chief symptom, followed by gastrointestinal and respiratory disturbances. Symptoms were observed in the following order of frequency: irritability, tremors, vomiting, high pitched cry, sneezing, hypertonicity and hyperactivity, respiratory distress, fever, diarrhea, mucus secretion, and sweating. Chlorpromazine was used for treating 46.3%. Mortality was 3.6%. There was no increase in congenital anomalies.

CONCLUSIONS

The complications observed may relate to addiction, but may also relate to nutritional deprivation, inadequate prenatal care, and low socio-economic status. Special programs for early case finding and total socio-medical support are needed. Methadone detoxification regimens appear promising. The authors recommend withdrawing and detoxifying patients during pregnancy and post-partum.

The high incidence of low birth weight raises the possibility that narcotic use may cause intrauterine growth retardation, but long-term effects are difficult to determine. The authors feel strongly that obstetricians and pediatricians should become familiar with the problems of pregnant addicts and the symptoms of neonates, so that proper treatment can result in improved perinatal outcome.

Stern, Roy. The pregnant addict: A study of 66 case histories, 1950-1959. American Journal of Obstetrics and Gynecology, 94: 253-257, January 1966.

DRUG	Opiates
SAMPLE SIZE	66 Mothers; 70 Neonates
SAMPLE TYPE	Treatment (inpatient)
AGE	Neonates
SEX	Not Specified
ETHNICITY	Not Specified
GEOGRAPHICAL AREA	Metropolitan Hospital, New York, New York
METHODOLOGY	Case Studies
DATA COLLECTION INSTRUMENT	Laboratory/Examination; Program/ Clinic Statistics
DATE(S) CONDUCTED	Dates of Records Studied: 1950-1959
NO. OF REFERENCES	2

SUMMARY

Case histories of 66 pregnant narcotic addicts were analyzed to determine the problems and complications of pregnancies in this group. It was found that this group averaged less than one prenatal visit per patient; that 40.9% showed obstetrical complications; and that the median number of years of addiction was approximately 5 years. The author suggests additional efforts for this population including a multiple team of pediatrician and psychiatrist during early pregnancy.

METHODOLOGY

The sample consisted of 66 consecutive cases from the records of the Metropolitan Health Center. Pregnancies were analyzed for obstetrical history, complications of current pregnancy and narcotics addiction. The figures compiled were statistically analyzed for significance of variance from the general population at that medical center.

FINDINGS

Obstetrical Complications

Twenty-seven (40. 9%) addicted mothers showed toxemia, abruptio placentae, retained placenta, postpartum hemorrhage, ruptured marginal sinus cephalopelvic disproportion, and breech presentation. Toxemia of pregnancy (15. 1%), abruptio placental (9%), and postpartum hemorrhage (9%) were high compared to the general population of the same hospital. Breech presentations constituted 12% of the cases as compared with 4. 8% for the hospital in general.

Newborn Information

A highly significant incidence of prematurity (18. 5%) was noted versus 8. 6% in the general population. There were 57 term deliveries, 13 premature and 5 stillborn. Stillborns constituted 7. 1% of the addicted group as compared to 2. 9% of the general hospital population.

Medical Complications

Of the 40 cases in which the serology was known, 20% were positive. Other medical complications noted on admission to the hospital were multiple abscesses, cellulitis, venous thrombosis, and serum hepatitis.

CONCLUSIONS

Chances of toxemia are significantly greater among addicts; placental abnormalities are more frequent; breech presentations occur more often; and postpartum hemorrhage is more likely. There is nothing to indicate that labor is prolonged in the addict. The infant of the addict is more likely to be premature and/or stillborn.

Because of the lack of prenatal care and the conditions of environmental and poor health care the addict is subject to, no conclusion can be made as to the actual cause of complications.

The greatest difficulties in these cases occur after delivery for both infant and mother. Twenty percent of the patients in this study left the hospital against advice, presumably to obtain heroin to offset withdrawal symptoms.

Zelson, Carl; Rubio, Estrellita; and Wasserman, Edward. Neonatal narcotic addiction: Ten year observation. Pediatrics, 48(2):178-189, August, 1971.

DRUG	Opiates
SAMPLE SIZE	384
SAMPLE TYPE	Treatment (inpatient)
AGE	Infants
SEX	Both Male and Female
ETHNICITY	Not Specified
GEOGRAPHICAL AREA	New York, New York
METHODOLOGY	Case Studies
DATA COLLECTION INSTRUMENT	Observations; Laboratory/Examination
DATE(S) CONDUCTED	1960-1969
NO. OF REFERENCES	20

SUMMARY

A group of infants born to heroin addicted mothers was observed during a 10 year period at New York Medical College, Metropolitan Hospital Center. The identification of the mother as a narcotic addict was based on the history taken by the admitting physician and confirmed by repeated patient interviews and by evidence found on examination, i.e., needle marks, scars, and so forth. The infants were observed and followed during their stay in the hospital. Considerable variation in the clinical course was observed from infant to infant. All infants of these mothers developed symptoms which were mild with low maternal heroin dosage, and severe with high maternal dosage. Severity of symptoms, time of onset, and duration of symptoms were found to be related to the size of maternal heroin dosage, to the length of maternal drug addiction, and to the time the last dose was taken.

METHODOLOGY

During the years 1960 through 1969, a total of 384 infants born to 382 heroin addicted mothers was observed and followed by the authors during their entire stay in the hospital. Infants with minimal or mild withdrawal signs were not treated. The untreated or control group was compared with the treated group as well as with nonaddicted infants.

FINDINGS

Of the 384 infants born to 382 heroin addicted mothers, 190 (49.4%) of the infants were under 2,500 gm in weight. Seventy-seven (40%) of these were low weight for date infants. Two hundred fifty-nine (67.4%) of the total group of infants developed signs of withdrawal within the first 4 days of life. One hundred seventy-eight or 68.7% of these manifested signs severe enough to require treatment. Eighty-one infants had mild withdrawal signs which cleared without treatment. The 178 treated infants represented 46.3% of the entire group of heroin exposed infants. A total of 14 infants died, a 3.6% mortality rate. Congenital abnormalities did not occur with any more frequency than in the general population.

The data in this study indicate:

1. The incidence of infant withdrawal syndrome was higher in the group of mothers on high drug doses.

2. There was a direct correlation between time and frequency of the onset of withdrawal signs in the infants, and the time span between the mother's last dose of drug and the birth of the infant.

3. The longer the mother was on drugs, the higher was the incidence of withdrawal in the newborn infants.

No correlation could be established between dosage taken by the mother and the occurrence of low birth weight infants. Morphine and/or quinine was shown to be present in the urine of newborn infants of addicted mothers within the first 24 hours after birth. The presence of morphine or quinine did not necessarily indicate that the infant would develop withdrawal signs. The incidence of hyperbilirubinemia was lower than occurs in the general newborn population.

CONCLUSIONS

Three reasons are suggested to explain why one-third of the infants born to heroin-addicted mothers do not develop withdrawal, or why some who do have signs of withdrawal do not show evidence of withdrawal: (1) the drug does not get across the placenta; (2) it may cross the placenta in too small amounts, or (3) the infant does not respond to the drug unless a metabolic change has occurred to trigger the onset of signs.

The authors believe that maternal narcotic addiction seriously affects the fetus and has a damaging effect on the newborn infant. The incidence of reaction of withdrawal is quite high and mortality may also be high if the condition is not recognized and treated. Early recognition and treatment of infants of drug addicted mothers will significantly reduce the mortality rate among these infants.

Schulman, Carol A. Alterations of the sleep cycle in heroin-addicted and "suspect" newborns. Neuropaediatrie, 1:89-100, June-July, 1969.

DRUG	Heroin
SAMPLE SIZE	24
SAMPLE TYPE	Treatment (inpatient)
AGE	Neonates
SEX	Not Specified
ETHNICITY	Not Specified
GEOGRAPHICAL AREA	New York City
METHODOLOGY	Controlled/Experimental
DATA COLLECTION INSTRUMENT	Observations
DATE(S) CONDUCTED	Not Specified
NO. OF REFERENCES	10

SUMMARY

The sleep cycle of normal newborns consists of 2 regularly alternating phases, active sleep and quiet sleep, each characterized by
distinctive EEG patterns, heart rate, EMG, and eye movements.
The purpose of this study was to examine the extent of deviations
from this norm in the sleep cycle of newborns in whom perinatal
events affecting the central nervous system (CNS) had occurred.
If conditions which affect the CNS have a direct effect on the sleep
cycle, then the relationship of this cycle and the effects of heroin
withdrawal at birth can be studied.

The frequency of rapid eye movements (REMS) in infants with
suspicion of CNS impairment was also examined. Analyses of
the polygraphic records of 8 normal control, 8 CNS high risk, and
8 infants born to heroin-addicted mothers showed that both experimental groups deviated markedly from the control, exhibiting
dissociation of the variables that characterize the normal sleep
cycle. Newborns with CNS impairment had higher resting levels
of activity. Quiet sleep, as usually defined, did not develop,
although there were cyclic changes in activity level as a function
of changing EEG activity. The heroin-addicted newborns showed
the greatest disturbance.

METHODOLOGY

The subjects chosen were all healthy, full-term infants aged 3-14
days. None had abnormal EEG's. None had been given any medication since birth. There were 3 groups of 8 subjects each:
a normal control group; a CNS risk group composed of newborns
with a variety of fetal or neurological distresses; and a group
born to heroin-addicted mothers which showed signs of primary
withdrawal, but which also evidenced clear abatement of the withdrawal before inclusion in the study.

Electrodes to record EEG, EKG, and EMG signals were affixed
after the 10 a.m. feeding. The infant was then permitted to fall
asleep. No further intervention occurred until the end of the
recording period. Recording ended only when a period of quiet
sleep had been superseded by a well-established period of active
sleep, or after 45 minutes if there had been no noticeable change.
All data were based on the first 45 minutes of recording, which
was the first sleep cycle after the midmorning feeding. The recordings were supplemented by behavioral observations, which
were used to determine periods of wakefulness, drowsiness or
crying. Such periods were excluded from analysis.

FINDINGS

Analysis of the results showed significant departures from the
normal sleep pattern in both experimental groups. All normal
newborns displayed the classic sleep pattern of active sleep
accompanied by low voltage fast wave (LVFW) EEG activity, frequent body movements, variable heart rate, frequent REMS alternating with quiet sleep accompanied by high voltage slow wave
(HVSW) EEG activity, absence of body or eye movements, and
a generally regular heart rate.

The normal cycle, alternating between active and quiet sleep, was absent in the experimental subjects. Active sleep was accompanied by greater activity in all variables, while quiet sleep did not develop. However, all subjects showed cyclic changes in activity level which coincided with EEG voltage changes. On REMS and body movement variables, heroin addicted subjects showed the greatest sleep disturbance, and time spent in HVSW sleep was more variable.

CONCLUSIONS

Results indicate that the sleep cycle of a newborn infant is a highly sensitive indicator of the presence of events which affect CNS. The data suggest that resting activity levels are high in newborns exposed to conditions which affect CNS unfavorably.

Blinick, George; Tavolga, William N.; and Antopol, William.
Variations in birth cries of newborn infants from narcotic-addicted
and normal mothers. American Journal of Obstetrics and Gynecology,
110(7):948-958, August 1, 1971.

DRUG	Opiates
SAMPLE SIZE	369
SAMPLE TYPE	Treatment (inpatient)
AGE	369 Neonates
SEX	Not Specified
ETHNICITY	Not Specified
GEOGRAPHICAL AREA	New York, New York
METHODOLOGY	Comparative
DATA COLLECTION INSTRUMENT	Laboratory/Examination
DATE(S) CONDUCTED	Not Specified
NO. OF REFERENCES	13

SUMMARY

This study compared the birth cries of neonates born to normal and
addicted mothers. Many clinicians claim that the birth cry of the
neonate born of an addicted mother is characteristic and recognizable.
It is described as a high-pitched, piercing, and continuous cry which
is heard from birth to 60 minutes or longer after delivery. The neonate's vocalization is a valid index of physiologic condition. This investigation recorded the birth cries of neonates and analyzed them on a
purely physical acoustic basis. The questions asked were: (1) What
are the normal acoustic parameters of the neonate vocalization?

(2) What variations in these parameters occur in a normal population sample? (3) What variations can be considered abnormal or pathologic? (4) Can such abnormal variations be correlated with maternal drug addiction? (5) What is the potential value of such acoustic analysis as a diagnostic tool?

METHODOLOGY

The data consisted of tape recordings of birth cries of infants delivered at Beth Israel Hospital. A total of 369 cases were recorded and analyzed, of which 31 were infants born of drug-addicted mothers. Recordings were made in the delivery room, within moments of birth, and, in most cases, the very first vocalizations were included. The recorded samples averaged about 3 minutes, and several cases of a continuous 20 minute sample were included. For each sample, the first several vocalizations that were clearly recorded were selected for spectrographic analysis, and the entire sample was monitored aurally. Occasionally, some of the sounds appearing later in the sample were also analyzed.

Based upon 338 recorded cases of birth from non-drug-addicted mothers, 145 were chosen as representing normal vocalization, with no indications of any pathologic conditions in the case history. "Typical" birth cries and common variants of the normal birth cry were listed and described, including variations in duration, intensity, quality and pitch. Of the 369 cases, 53 were judged to be abnormal. Variations in pitch, quality and other parameters were distinct and the variations were consistently present throughout the recorded sample. A schema for classification of infant vocalization was adopted as the first step in the utilization of the spectrograms as well as other methods in identifying significant characteristics of the sounds.

FINDINGS

It was evident that there was a considerable amount of variation in the acoustic characteristics of human birth cries, even among vocalizations emitted by the same individual over a period of a few minutes. One function of this report was to demonstrate the degree of this variation in normal individuals and to determine what parameters of the sounds were measurable and significant. The kinds of variations that fall within the normal range consisted primarily of differences in the degree of nonharmonic distortion. Variations in fundamental frequency tended to be less variable within the individual, and extremely high or low frequencies were classified as abnormal. The abnormality most characteristic of infants from drug-addicted mothers seemed to be a high-pitched, squealing cry. Furthermore, the data showed clearly that the percentage of extreme abnormalities was higher among the drug-addicted cases.

CONCLUSIONS

On the basis of the data given here, it is clear that some relationship exists between abnormalities in birth cries of the neonate and
the drug addiction of the mother. This reinforces the validity of the
use of birth cries as a general diagnostic tool. Acoustic analysis
of tape recordings by means of a sound spectrograph is valuable in
preserving the data and making quantitative analysis possible. The
spectrograph is already established as a standard tool in human
speech analysis and can certainly be utilized in the investigation of
infant vocalizations. The qualitative evaluations of the physician
in the delivery room should be considered as an essential part of
the recorded data, along with spectrographic and other analyses.

Glass, L; Rajegowda, B.K.; Kahn, E.J.; and Floyd, M.V.
Effect of heroin withdrawal on respiratory rate and acid-base status
in the newborn. New England Journal of Medicine, 286(14):746-748,
April 6, 1972.

DRUG	Heroin
SAMPLE SIZE	41
SAMPLE TYPE	Treatment (inpatient)
AGE	Neonates
SEX	Not Specified
ETHNICITY	Not Specified
GEOGRAPHICAL AREA	New York City
METHODOLOGY	Comparative
DATA COLLECTION INSTRUMENT	Laboratory/Examination
DATE(S) CONDUCTED	December 1970 - April 1971
NO. OF REFERENCES	14

SUMMARY

The study was made to demonstrate high respiratory rates in newborn infants with heroin-withdrawal symptoms and their effect on
acid-base status. Measurements of respiratory rates and acid-
base status were made on 22 infants born to addict mothers and 19
normal infants of similar weight and gestational age. The infants
experiencing heroin withdrawal manifested increased respiratory
rates associated with hypocapnia and an increase in blood pH during
the first week after birth.

The observed respiratory alkalosis may play a beneficial role in binding indirect serum bilirubin to albumin. It may prevent respiratory-distress syndrome, but alkalosis decreases the levels of ionized calcium.

METHODOLOGY

Data were obtained from 22 infants with withdrawal symptoms, and 19 infants born to non-addicts, at Harlem Hospital, between December 1970, and April 1971. Addicted infants were selected on the basis of maternal history of addiction, symptoms of irritability, and coarse flapping tremors. Other withdrawal symptoms were also frequently present.

Birth weight ranged from 1220 to 3370 gm. (median 2070 gm.). Gestational age ranged from 32 to 40 weeks (median 37 weeks). None of the infants were obviously ill nor was there evidence of respiratory-distress, meconium aspiration, anemia or polycythemia, infection or hyperpyrexia. Withdrawal symptoms began within 24 hours for 19 infants, and persisted for 2 to 6 days. Sixteen infants were treated with phenobarbital.

The birth weight of the randomly selected control infants ranged from 1250 to 4400 gm. (median 1980 gm.); gestational age ranged from 32 to 40 weeks (median 36). Both groups were kept in the same type of incubators at the same temperature, and fed orally with Enfamil. Respiratory rates were counted 4 times per day and tabulated to determine the daily mean. Measurements were taken of blood pH and carbon dioxide tension (P_{CO_2}) of all infants on the first through fourth days of life. Additional analyses on half of subjects were taken on the fifth and seventh days, and on five subjects in each group during the second week of life.

FINDINGS

Infants with heroin-withdrawal symptoms had significantly higher respiratory rates during the first week. P_{CO_2} levels were significantly lower; blood pH was elevated significantly on the second, third, and fourth days. During the second week differences were less noticeable. Findings were independent of birth weight, gestational age, or severity of symptoms. Respiratory rate was not influenced by phenobarbital use.

CONCLUSIONS

Diagnosis of heroin withdrawal presently relies on unquantifiable observations (crying, irritability). Their findings suggest that an accurate count of respiration may prove to be a more precise diagnostic procedure. However, the hyperpnea of withdrawal is difficult to observe because addicted infants are rarely still, and because brief bursts of rapid respiration occur among normal neonates. The cause of hyperpnea is unknown. In adult addicts it is attributed to increased sensitivity to carbon dioxide.

Hyperventilation may have beneficial effects in newborn infants. Despite the high incidence of low birth weight and premature gestational age, respiratory-distress syndrome is very rare. The elevated blood pH may protect against pulmonary hypoperfusion; it may also reduce risk from bilirubin encephalopathy, since bilirubin binding capacity of albumin improves with a rising pH.

However, the possible causative relation between low ionized calcium levels and the jerks or seizures requires further study.

Klain, David B.; Krauss, Alfred N.; and Auld, Peter A. M.
Tachypnea and alkalosis in infants of narcotic-addicted mothers.
New York State Journal of Medicine, 72(3):367-368, February 1,
1972.

DRUG	Heroin
SAMPLE SIZE	9
SAMPLE TYPE	Treatment (inpatient)
AGE	Neonates
SEX	Not Specified
ETHNICITY	Not Specified
GEOGRAPHICAL AREA	New York, New York
METHODOLOGY	Case Studies
DATA COLLECTION INSTRUMENT	Laboratory/Examination
DATE(S) CONDUCTED	Not Specified
NO. OF REFERENCES	9

SUMMARY

This report presents data on 9 newborn infants of heroin-addicted
mothers. Tachypnea and respiratory alkalosis were noted in these
infants; it is suggested that this abnormal state is an explanation of
some of the symptoms frequently exhibited by infants of narcotic-
addicted mothers.

METHODOLOGY

Arterial blood gases were measured. Blood samples were taken from
the temporal artery in 8 cases, the femoral artery in 1.

Determinations of pH and carbon dioxide and oxygen pressures were made immediately after sampling and results were corrected to the infant's body temperature.

Blood glucose was measured by the Glucostat enzyme method and calcium by atomic absorption spectrophotometry.

Patients had no clinical or radiologic evidence of hyaline membrane disease and were breathing room air when studied.

FINDINGS

All but 1 infant demonstrated respiratory alkalosis when compared with normal arterial pH and blood gas values.

All were symptomatic, and all except 1 demonstrated tachypnea.

Blood glucose and serum calcium values (except 1) were normal. The exception had a blood sugar of 15 at 3 hours of age.

Among the 9 infants, birth weights ranged from 1,620-3,520 grams; gestational age ranged from 31-40 weeks; the onset of symptoms appeared between 24 and 48 hours after birth. Mothers had received their last dose of heroin from 1.5 to 72 hours prior to delivery.

CONCLUSIONS

Alkalosis in infants of addicted mothers suggests that some of the symptoms may be directly related to a disturbance in acid-base metabolism. Such a conclusion would reinforce the theory that tetany of alkalosis is attributed to an alteration of ionized calcium.

Naeye, Richard L., et al. Fetal complications of maternal heroin addiction: Abnormal growth, infections, and episodes of stress. The Journal of Pediatrics, 83(6):1055-1061, December, 1973.

DRUG	Heroin
SAMPLE SIZE	95
SAMPLE TYPE	Treatment (inpatient) and Incarcerated
AGE	Neonates
SEX	54 Male and 41 Female
ETHNICITY	65 Black, 15 Puerto Rican, 14 White
GEOGRAPHICAL AREA	New York City
METHODOLOGY	Case Study
DATA COLLECTION INSTRUMENT	Laboratory/Examination Program/Clinic Statistics
DATE(S) CONDUCTED	1954 to 1972
NO. OF REFERENCES	34

SUMMARY

Eighty-two drug-addicted women who used heroin throughout pregnancy and their neonates were examined. Nearly 60% of the mothers or their newborn infants had evidence of acute infection. Most of the infected mothers delivered prematurely, whereas those not infected delivered at term. Meconium histiocytosis was very common in the placentas of heroin-exposed infants, suggesting that they had experienced episodes of distress during fetal life. As a group, infants born to heroin addicts were small for gestational age; all organs were affected. Retardation of fetal growth could not always be explained by undernutrition of the addicted mother.

METHODOLOGY

Medical records were examined of 59 neonates born to addict mothers between 1954 and 1972 at the Columbia-Presbyterian Medical Center in New York City. All mothers used heroin up to the time of delivery. Control subjects were 500 consecutive infants born at the same medical center.

Postmortem material from Harlem and Bellevue Hospitals was also examined: 23 live newborn and stillborn infants of addicted mothers. These mothers also used heroin up to the time of delivery.

Other postmortem cases included 10 neonates whose mothers used heroin only in the early months of pregnancy; these mothers were in prisons or other institutions during the last trimester of gestation.

Autopsy data were included from 7 infants whose nonaddicted mothers had clinical features of hepatitis during or before pregnancy.

Additional control subjects included 1,044 consecutive autopsies performed on well-preserved stillborn and newborn infants at Babies Hospital.

Hospital records were used to obtain organ and body weights and measurements. Planimetry, line sampling and point counting were used to quantitate the volume of individual components in the various organs. These methods were also used to determine the relative sizes and numbers of cells and cellular components in the various organs. Chi squares and Students' t tests were used to determine the significance of various data.

FINDINGS

Maternal nutrition (body weight before pregnancy and weight gain during pregnancy) was found to be the major factor influencing fetal growth, independent of the mother's interval since last pregnancy, height, race, age, occupation, economic or marital status. Thirty-six mothers addicted to heroin throughout their pregnancies were classified as over- or underweight soon after conception and were monitored to parturition. The infants born to the heroin addicts showed growth retardation regardless of the mother's weight gain. The underweight condition in these infants differed from that found in the infants of nonaddicts: there was a decreased number of cells in the organs of the infants (rather than simply smaller organs, as found in the latter cases).

Other explanations of retarded fetal growth in heroin addicts included deficient growth hormones and episodes of withdrawal, which may cause fetal distress. Even though half of all heroin addicts

are known to have hepatitis, this disease was not a factor in fetal
retardation since fetuses exposed to hepatitis by nonaddict mothers
evidenced no growth abnormalities. Addicted mothers with clinical features of infection delivered prematurely, while non-infected
addicts delivered full term infants.

CONCLUSIONS

The adrenal cortisol released by the infected fetuses may be responsible for initiating early labor; however, there is a "beneficial"
side effect of accelerating lung maturation and thus reducing the
incidence of hyaline membrane disease in these infants.

Although no conclusions were drawn from this study about the
teratogenicity of heroin, it was noted that other agents which
reduce cellular multiplication (such as rubella) are known to be
teratogenic.

Glass, Leonard; Rajegowda, B.K.; and Evans, Hugh E. Absence of respiratory distress syndrome in premature infants of heroin-addicted mothers. Lancet, 2:685-686, September 25, 1971.

DRUG	Heroin
SAMPLE SIZE	156
SAMPLE TYPE	Treatment (inpatient)
AGE	Neonates
SEX	Both Male and Female
ETHNICITY	Not Specified
GEOGRAPHICAL AREA	New York City
METHODOLOGY	Comparative
DATA COLLECTION INSTRUMENT	Program/Clinic Statistics
DATE(S) CONDUCTED	1971
NO. OF REFERENCES	8

SUMMARY

A comparison of infants born prematurely to both heroin-addicted and nonheroin-addicted mothers showed no cases of respiratory distress syndrome (R.D.S.) in the former as opposed to 26 cases of R.D.S. in the latter.

A previous study found that infants with symptoms of heroin withdrawal systematically demonstrated a respiratory alkalosis beginning on the first day of life. The effects of this are not yet understood, nor is it known whether opiates stimulate surfactant, an enzyme whose absence has been linked to R.D.S.

METHODOLOGY

A retrospective comparison was made of 156 pre-term infants of
37 weeks gestation or less, to determine the prevalence of R. D. S.
Patients had been admitted to the special care nursery of Harlem
Hospital Center between January 1968 and May 1971.

Heroin withdrawal in infants was diagnosed as coarse tremors,
irritability and a shrill high-pitched cry.

Diagnosis of R. D. S. was based on the presence of chest retraction, grunting, cyanosis in room air and absence of any other
recognized cause for respiratory distress such as pneumonia or
pneumothorax.

FINDINGS

It was found that R. D. S. was generally mild and transient if the
infant was 34 weeks or older, and more severe if younger than
34 weeks. Three deaths occurred in the 32-33 weeks group; one
death in the 34-35 week group; the 36-37 week cases all survived.
There were no cases of R. D. S. among the infants born to heroin-
addicted mothers, nor any deaths in that group.

CONCLUSIONS

R. D. S. is rare in neonates born to heroin-addicted mothers
regardless of gestational age. Heroin-addicted infants may have
a protective mechanism against R. D. S. The authors suggest
that opiates may function as enzyme inducers resulting in accel-
erated production of surfactant, whose absence or decreased
presence in the lungs of pre-term babies had been linked to R. D. S.
Further studies are indicated.

Behrendt, Hans, and Green, Marvin.   Nature of the sweating deficit of prematurely born neonates: Observations on babies with the heroin withdrawal syndrome. The New England Journal of Medicine, 286(26):1376-1379, June 26, 1972.

DRUG	Heroin
SAMPLE SIZE	259
SAMPLE TYPE	Treatment (inpatient)
AGE	Neonates
SEX	Not Specified
ETHNICITY	Not Specified
GEOGRAPHICAL AREA	New York City
METHODOLOGY	Controlled/Experimental
DATA COLLECTION INSTRUMENT	Laboratory/Examination
DATE(S) CONDUCTED	Not Specified
NO. OF REFERENCES	19

SUMMARY

The study examined the frequency of spontaneous background sweating among addicted, as well as healthy, low-birth-weight infants, and healthy full-sized infants.

Thirty of 131 healthy, full-sized, and two of 108 newborn, infants manifested spontaneous generalized sweating under standardized conditions, in contrast to 8 of 20 low-birth-weight infants of heroin addicts.

The pharmacologic threshold for sweating was decreased in the low-birth-weight addicted infants compared to the healthy low-birth-weight control group. The authors concluded that this paradox may be due to predominantly central neurogenic stimulation of sweat glands induced by heroin withdrawal.

All infants were aged between 1 and 8 days. All were kept at controlled temperatures (31° to $34^\circ C$ for low birth weight, 29° to $31^\circ C$ for full size) in incubators; they were observed for generalized sweating during a 2 hour adaptation period and during the actual performance of intradermal stimulation tests.

Generalized sweating was tested using the Wada modification of the starch iodine reaction, or by sweat prints on bromphenol blue paper applied to the skin.

Local sweating reaction to intradermally injected epinephrine, acetylcholine, and nicotine, under similarly controlled thermal conditions, was also observed. Positive response was noted if at least five sweat spots could be seen after ten minutes. The minimal effect concentration was determined for each drug. The strongest solution used was 1.0 mg. per milliliter for epinephrine and acetylcholine, and 0.1 mg. per milliliter for nicotine.

FINDINGS

The frequency of generalized sweating for healthy full size infants, over 2,500 g. birth weight, and 39 to 42 weeks of gestational age, was 30 out of 131. For healthy, low birth weight (936-2,466 g.), and 27-39 weeks of gestational age, the frequency was 2 out of 108. For addicted low-birth-weight infants (907-2,390 g.), also 27-39 weeks, the frequency was 8 out of 20. Only addicted infants manifested actual hyperhidrosis. Sweating occurred when they were at complete rest.

Comparative responsiveness (threshold) to intradermal pharmacologic stimulation was tested using 3 paired groups of healthy and addicted infants. In each of the paired groups, many infants failed to sweat in response to the most concentrated drug solution. Thus, evaluation must be based on comparative proportions. The proportion of infants with measurable thresholds was found significantly higher among addicted than control infants in tests with all 3 drugs. Sweat glands of addicted infants developed abnormally high reactivity to direct stimulation as the result of drug withdrawal. Threshold concentrations tended to decrease with increasing gestational age, and were exaggerated in the addicted infants.

CONCLUSIONS

Generalized sweating is of central neurogenic origin, which is
deficient in the normal premature infant. The addicted premature
infant's sweating mechanism is activated under the influence of
withdrawal to an efficiency equal to, or more than, that of full term
newborns.

The pathophysiologic disturbances of the withdrawal syndrome
product increased tonicity of the sweat fibers, providing tonic
innervation which sustains glandular reactivity and makes the end
organ susceptible to direct pharmacologic stimulation. The second
effect is generation of actual nerve impulses that create the conditions for thermal reflex sweating and hyperhidrosis. The increased glandular responsiveness associated with the withdrawal
syndrome cannot be explained by the law of denervation.

The authors conclude that in healthy premature infants, the central
and glandular components of sweating lack responsiveness, but
the end organ is potentially operative. Its reactivity depends on
central autonomic output. Heroin withdrawal is an example of
a central nervous disorder which leads to hyperactivity of the
sweating centers. Functional maturation of the sweat response at
birth depends on an intact cerebral innervation during development
in utero.

Hill, R. M. , and Desmond, M. M. Management of the narcotic
withdrawal syndrome in the neonate. Pediatric Clinics of
North America, 10:67-86, February 1963.

DRUG	Heroin
SAMPLE SIZE	4
SAMPLE TYPE	Treatment (inpatient)
AGE	4 Neonates
SEX	2 Male; 2 Female
ETHNICITY	4 White
GEOGRAPHICAL AREA	Houston, Texas
METHODOLOGY	Case Study
DATA COLLECTION INSTRUMENT	Laboratory/Examination
DATE(S) CONDUCTED	Not Specified
NO. OF REFERENCES	38

SUMMARY

Female narcotic addicts are typically malnourished women with poor
standards of self-care. When they are pregnant, prenatal care is
not sought, and they frequently arrive at the hospital in active labor.
On admission, the majority of narcotic addicts do not give a history
of addiction, therefore the physician's suspicion should be aroused if
the usual amount of analgesic does not ease the pains of labor. In
general, from 83 to 91 percent of infants born to actively addicted
mothers will manifest withdrawal symptoms within the first day of
life. The mortality rate has been reported to range between 34 and
93 percent, with the greatest mortality occurring within the first two

weeks of life. The oldest form of therapy for addicted infants is to have them breast fed by mothers. Paregoric has been frequently employed in dosages ranging from 5 to 10 drops every 10 minutes to 20 drops every 4 hours. The dose is gradually reduced after one to three weeks of therapy. The successful use of methadone in the gradual detoxification of narcotic addicted infants has also been reported; a dosage of 0.5 mg. every 4 to 12 hours produced no toxic effects. In addition barbiturates (typically phenobarbital), reserpine and chlorpromazine have also been employed to allay withdrawal signs. Several case histories of addicted infants and their management regimens are presented.

Kahn, Eric J.; Neumann, Lois L.; and Polk, Gene-Ann. The course of the heroin withdrawal syndrome in newborn infants treated with phenobarbital or chlorpromazine. The Journal of Pediatrics, 75(3):495-500, September, 1969.

DRUG	Heroin, Chlorpromazine, Phenobarbital
SAMPLE SIZE	38
SAMPLE TYPE	Treatment (inpatient)
AGE	38 neonates
SEX	Not Specified
ETHNICITY	Not Specified
GEOGRAPHICAL AREA	New York City
METHODOLOGY	Controlled/Experimental
DATA COLLECTION INSTRUMENT	Laboratory/Examination
DATE(S) CONDUCTED	October 1966 to September 1967
NO. OF REFERENCES	13

SUMMARY

A double-blind study was conducted at two New York hospitals using phenobarbital and chlorpromazine in the treatment of heroin withdrawal syndrome in infants, in order to assess the relative efficacy of each drug and the possible development of habituation to chlorpromazine.

METHODOLOGY

Thirty-eight infants born to heroin-addicted mothers manifested the withdrawal symptoms of tremors (all 38), irritability (33 of 38), shrill cry (21 of 38), muscle rigidity (17 of 38), and skin abrasions from excessive movement (14 of 38). The infants having tremors and irritability (the most reliable indicators of heroin withdrawal syndrome) were divided into three groups according to the severity of their symptoms.

The infants were then assigned at random to treatment groups as follows:

Number of Infants	Group	Dosage
12	PS(phenobarbital, short course)	8.4 mg/kg/day, in 4 doses/day for 4 days
7	PL (phenobarbital, long course)	Same dose as PS for ten days; then reduced 1/3 each 48 hrs. to 16 days
11	CS(chlorpromazine, short course)	2.8 mg/kg/day, in 4 doses/day for 4 days
8	CL (chlorpromazine, long course)	Same dose as CS for ten days, gradually reduced for next 6 days

The drugs were dispensed in a syrup base so that equal volumes supplied the standard dose of either drug; in this way, drug identification was impossible to the observers who would note the changes in the intensity of the infants' symptoms.

RESULTS

One infant died of unknown causes at 1 1/2 months after having recovered from withdrawal symptoms at 3 days of age. There were no other deaths, but diarrhea and vomiting were noted in some infants as prognostically adverse factors. No other serious complications were evidenced in this study.

Thirty of the infants became asymptomatic after 4 days of treatment. Eight infants, 6 of them in the short treatment group, showed symptoms beyond 4 days, but in all cases their degree of improvement precluded the resumption of medication.

No dependence on either chlorpromazine or phenobarbital was noted at the termination of the long course groups.

CONCLUSIONS

In assessing the desirability of one drug over the other, it was noted that myoclonus occurred less frequently with phenobarbital, but due to the absence of a control group (for humane reasons) no conclusions could be drawn about the relative length of recovery periods.

Nathenson, Gerald; Golden, Gerald S.; and Litt, Iris F.
Diazepam in the management of the neonatal narcotic withdrawal
syndrome. Pediatrics, 48(4):523-527, October, 1971.

DRUG	Diazepam (Valium)
SAMPLE SIZE	18
SAMPLE TYPE	Parent-Child, Treatment (inpatient) Treatment (outpatient)
AGE	Neonates
SEX	10 Male and 8 Female
ETHNICITY	Not Specified
GEOGRAPHICAL AREA	Bronx, New York
METHODOLOGY	Experimental
DATA COLLECTION INSTRUMENT	Laboratory/Examination
DATE(S) CONDUCTED	1969 to 1970
NO. OF REFERENCES	30

SUMMARY

Diazepam (Valium) was administered intramuscularly to 18 infants
born of mothers addicted to heroin. This drug appeared to be a
safe and effective treatment for neonatal heroin withdrawal symptoms. The course of therapy was short, and serious side effects
or rebound symptoms did not recur when treatment was discontinued.

METHODOLOGY

The stated intent of this report is to describe those observations which document the usefulness of diazepam (Valium) in the management of the neonatal withdrawal syndrome. Eighteen infants were observed during a 10-month period. The addicting drug in all pregnancies was heroin, but 1 mother was in a methadone treatment program. The infants were classified as mildly, moderately, or severely affected, based on clinical criteria observed within the first 48 hours of life. These criteria included measures of tremulousness, mild autonomic disorders, vomiting, diarrhea, and convulsions. Of the 18 infants, 2 were classified as mild, 12 moderate, and 3 as severe cases. One neonate was viewed as being hypocalcemic, rather than addicted.

The treatment procedure consisted of administering intramuscularly an initial dose of 1 to 2 mg. of diazepam, based on the severity of the withdrawal symptoms and the size of the infant. This dose was repeated every 8 hours until symptoms were fully controlled. Then the dose was decreased to one-half that initially used, and then rapidly tapered by increasing the interval between injections to 12 hours and lowering the dose level to 0.5 mg. Full neurologic evaluations were performed at least once daily using standardized neonatal neurologic evaluation forms.

FINDINGS

Tremulousness and irritability disappeared within 24 hours in the mildly affected babies. It had previously been observed that such symptoms persisted for 1 week or more in untreated infants. Those infants classified as moderate or severe, and placed on therapy, experienced rapid control of symptoms within a mean period of 44.9 hours following the initial administration of diazepam (range 24 to 72 hours). The average duration of therapy was 3.9 days (ranged 1 1/4 to 6 days).

Neurologic examinations were normal, except for those findings that were part of the withdrawal syndrome. Determinations of serum calcium, magnesium, and total proteins in 9 of the addicted infants before, during, and after therapy uniformly revealed normal results. No infant showed a recurrence of symptoms following the cessation of treatment, and control of diarrhea was not a problem. Transient sedation, the only side effect noted, abated after the elimination of one dose or a decrease in dose. After complete withdrawal following an overdose, symptoms promptly disappeared and further therapy proved unnecessary. No local irritation occurred at sites of injection.

CONCLUSIONS

Two possible explanations were offered for the abbreviated course of illness and the absence of rebound symptoms, given the relatively short course of treatment. First, there could have been a correction of the pharmacologic disturbance. Secondly, the metabolism of diazepam is such that a long-acting effect results from its continued administration. When discontinued after 3 to 4 days of administration, there was still some drug measurable in the blood 1 week later. Superiority of diazepam over previously used agents was not claimed because a concurrent controlled series was not performed. Benefits of the study were noted to be quick withdrawal and absence of side effects, with recommended dosages of diazepam.

IV.   METHADONE

Statzer, D. E., and Wardell, J. N. Heroin addiction during pregnancy.
American Journal of Obstetrics and Gynecology, 113(2):273-278,
May 15, 1972.

DRUG	Methadone; Opiates
SAMPLE SIZE	150 Women; 100 Infants
SAMPLE TYPE	Parent-Child
AGE	Infants; Adults
SEX	Both Male and Female
ETHNICITY	135 Black; 15 White
GEOGRAPHICAL AREA	Detroit, Michigan
METHODOLOGY	Longitudinal
DATA COLLECTION INSTRUMENT	Medical Examination
DATE(S) CONDUCTED	Not Specified
NO. OF REFERENCES	8

SUMMARY

In the past the heroin addict was believed to be relatively infertile
because long term ingestion of heroin by women generally resulted
in menstrual irregularity, oligo-ovulation, decreased libido; and
salpingitis and subsequent infertility after recourse to prostitution.
However, the increased use of drugs together with an increase in the
number of young, short-term addicts taking smaller amounts of heroin,
has been associated with a larger number of fertile female addicts
who have become pregnant. This study was conducted to provide
physiologic and psychosociologic data concerning the effects of drug
addiction and its treatment during pregnancy.

After maintenance on the smallest daily dose of methadone required to prevent withdrawal symptoms in 150 pregnant heroin addicts, results indicated that out of the 90 infants born, 72 exhibited evidence of withdrawal, with only 23 requiring treatment. Those mothers who received less methadone had infants who evidenced greater withdrawal, and no correlation was obtained between the severity of withdrawal symptoms and the amount or duration of methadone administration.

METHODOLOGY

The subjects for the study were 150 pregnant heroin addicts who were enrolled in a methadone maintenance program at Wayne State University clinic. Fifteen were white; 135 were black. Over 62 percent were less than 23 years old (range 16 to 37). A mean gravidity of 3 and a parity of 1 led the authors to conclude that many had had one or more prior abortions.

The subjects administered heroin to themselves by various routes: nasal, 63; intravenous, 49; both nasal and intravenous, 36; not recorded, 2. Only 49 (32.6 percent) had used the intravenous route exclusively. The majority (66.4 percent) preferred "snorting" and only occasionally resorted to intravenous injections. Because the strength of pure heroin varied even within different areas of the city, and Detroit street heroin was approximately 10 percent heroin, 10 percent quinine, and 80 percent milk sugar, the determination of the exact amounts used was considered very difficult. The female addicts averaged 30 dollars a day and 19 months of use, indicating to the authors a short-term low dose usage in the majority who became pregnant.

Because the fetal effects of an increasing amount of methadone were not known, blockade was not attempted. Instead a maintenance program with the use of the smallest daily dose of methadone which would prevent maternal withdrawal symptoms was selected for this study. Because of noted correlations with the previous daily dose of heroin, after some experience had been gained, it was possible to select a beginning dose of methadone which required little or no change to prevent withdrawal symptoms. The daily methadone dosage averaged 45 mg (range, 10 to 110 mg), and for 63 percent of the subjects the range was between 10 to 30 mg. Eleven required no methadone.

Patients were required to return daily for methadone, which was taken in the presence of a physician or nurse. Prenatal care was provided in the usual manner. Amniocentesis was carried out in 20 patients before and after administration of methadone.

FINDINGS

One hundred infants were delivered: 2 were stillborn, 2 died soon after birth (not seen as drug related), 6 were delivered elsewhere. Although 79 of the live-born infants were delivered after 38 weeks of gestation, 37 weighed less than 6 lbs. The authors found it difficult to determine whether these infants were premature or low-birth-weight term infants. However, it is noted in a discussion following the article, that even in patients who had high levels of nutrition supplied by the maternal and infant care program there were low-birth-weight infants. In this study premature infants accounted for 26 percent of the total of 90 infants, and 56 percent were under 6 lbs, 9 ounces.

Of the 90 infants delivered in their hospital, the authors noted withdrawal symptoms (vomiting, diarrhea, irritability, and poor feeding) in 72. Symptoms were mild in 49, and no treatment was given. Tincture of opium was given to 18, phenobarbital to 3, Benadryl to 1, and Donatal to 1. No correlation was seen between the severity of withdrawal symptoms and the amount or duration of methadone administration. The average length of hospital stay for the infants was 13 days.

Out of 40 infants, urinalysis identified 20 with quinine and none with heroin. All mothers of the above 20 infants excreted quinine or heroin in the urine within 2 weeks prior to delivery. Amniocenteses performed in 20 patients after 38 week's gestation found bilirubin levels significantly higher than the observed level for non-heroin users in the same week of gestation. Creatinine levels were below 2.0 mg. percent in this study, and over 2.0 mg. percent for non-heroin users. At least 20 percent of fetal cells contained cytoplasmic lepid which compared with fetuses of non-heroin users. No congenital abnormalities were seen.

CONCLUSIONS

Further studies were called for to determine the significance of the amniocenteses results. Other results indicated that a higher level of heroin use was a factor in the severely affected infant. Although the majority of the women continued to take heroin during the time of methadone treatment, the mothers who were less regular in their daily attendance, and who received less methadone, produced infants requiring treatment.

Because quinine was found in the urine of the newborn infants, the authors have begun studies to determine fetal renal and hepatic effects of heroine, quinine, and methadone in subhuman primates in an attempt to correlate the physiologic effects in the fetus.

Maslansky, Robert A.; Sukov, Richard; and Beaumont, Graham. Pregnancies in Methadone Maintained Mothers. A Preliminary Report. Minneapolis, Minn.: Mt. Sinai Hospital, 1971. (Published in the 1971 Proceedings of the National Conference on Methadone Maintenance). 6 pp.

DRUG	Methadone
SAMPLE SIZE	4
SAMPLE TYPE	Treatment (inpatient)
AGE	1 Fetal, 3 Infants, 4 Adults (19-36)
SEX	Infants: 2 Male, 2 Female
ETHNICITY	1 Black, 3 White
GEOGRAPHICAL AREA	Minneapolis, Minnesota
METHODOLOGY	Case Studies
DATA COLLECTION INSTRUMENT	Laboratory/Examination
DATE(S) CONDUCTED	1971
NO. OF REFERENCES	14

SUMMARY

The pharmacology of methadone as it relates to pregnancy and the neonate was studied in the case histories of 4 addicts participating in a Minneapolis methadone treatment program. Placental transfer was shown, but no teratogenic effect of this was observed. Withdrawal symptoms similar to those of infants born to narcotic addicted mothers were anticipated, but only minimal withdrawal activity, not requiring medication, was observed.

CASE STUDIES

For each of the 4 case histories, maternal addiction and obstetric history, labor and delivery, and infant hospital course were recorded.

Case I

A 25-year-old Caucasian female gravida IV, para 3-0-0-3, blood type O negative. Negative serology and pap smear. Two-year history of heroin use prior to admission to methadone program. A 2,355 gm. female infant was born at 36-38 weeks gestation by normal spontaneous vaginal delivery. From day 5 infant was irritable. On day 11 X-ray revealed evidence of minimal pneumonitis, and there was clinical suggestion of congestive heart failure, and a positive urine culture of E. Coli 10. Despite treatment, respiration continued at 110, and there was temperature spiking, excessive perspiration, crying, and thrashing of limbs. The infant gained weight on day 15, was discharged day 26. Urine obtained on day 17 for qualitative methadone analysis was negative. Infant continued to thrive.

Case II

A 25-year-old Caucasian female gravida 5, para 1-0-3-2, blood type A positive. Negative serology and pap smear. History of heroin use for 2 1/2 years prior to admission to the program. A 2,580 gm. male infant was born at 38-40 weeks gestation, labor induced, vaginal delivery. Baby had rapid respirations 2 hours after birth. X-ray was suggestive of pseudorespiratory distress syndrome; respiration decreased by 8 hours after birth. On day 3 baby appeared jaundiced and underwent 2 exchanges. Baby was vigorous and fed well but showed unusual irritability during the first 4 post-transfusion days. Baby was examined and discharged as normal on day 11, and continued to thrive.

Case III

A 19-year-old Caucasian female gravida 2, para 0-0-1-0, O positive. Began using heroin and LSD in first trimester of pregnancy, was admitted to methadone program at 22 weeks gestation. Near term had a positive VDRL but a later FTA was negative. A female 3,015 gm. infant was born at 38 weeks gestation by spontaneous vaginal delivery. Neonatal course was complicated by initial positive VDRL. Repeat VDRL and FTA were negative. Infant discharged as normal after one week. No withdrawal symptoms manifested.

Case IV

A 36-year-old Negro female gravida IV, para 3-0-0-3. Spontaneous rupture of membranes at 20 weeks required I.V. Underwent pitocin induction and vacuum curettage. Male infant measured 11 cm., no congenital abnormality. Patient had a 2-year history of heroin addiction, was receiving 80 mg. liquid methadone a day at time of abortion.

FINDINGS

Findings substantiated the observations of previous studies that narcotic and methadone usage during pregnancy is associated with delivery of low birth weight infants. There was an absence of any life threatening withdrawal activity. The 2 infants whose mothers received the highest dosage of methadone did demonstrate activity consistent with withdrawal symptoms.

Despite significant placental transfer and accumulation of methadone, no congenital malformations were present.

CONCLUSIONS

A transiently positive VDRL occurred in case III; the authors suggest further investigation of the role of methadone and/or liver disease as a cause for a biologic false positive serologic test for syphilis. The relationship of methadone to the other pathology shown by infants I and II remains undefined. The authors hope to follow the infants to determine any latent consequences.

Pierson, Paul S.; Howard, Patricia; Kleber, Herbert D. Sudden deaths in infants born to methadone-maintained addicts. <u>Journal of the American Medical Association,</u> 220(13):1733-1744, June 26, 1972.

DRUG	Methadone
SAMPLE SIZE	14
SAMPLE TYPE	Treatment (inpatient)
AGE	Neonates
SEX	Both Male and Female
ETHNICITY	Not Specified
GEOGRAPHICAL AREA	New Haven, Connecticut
METHODOLOGY	Case Studies
DATA COLLECTION INSTRUMENT	Laboratory/Examination Program/Clinic Statistics
DATE(S) CONDUCTED	1968-1971
NO. OF REFERENCES	7

SUMMARY

Two confirmed and one possible case of sudden and unexpected death in infants less than 3 months of age occurred in a group of 14 infants of mothers who received methadone for opiate addiction during part of their pregnancy.

The pregnant women all received daily doses of methadone (average dose between 40-60 mg.). Treatment time ranged from one month to eight months prior to delivery. The average birth weight of the 14 newborns was 2,600 gm. Only 3 weighed less than 2,000 gm.

Within 3 hours of birth all infants were hyperactive, jittery, or had a shrill cry. All but 3 required treatment for withdrawal symptoms. None of the infants was breast fed.

The 3 deaths in the group of 14 may or may not have been methadone related. Because of this high incidence of the "sudden infant death syndrome", the authors urge further research in view of the expansion of methadone maintenance programs.

CASE STUDIES

Case 1

The only infant to be given methadone immediately after birth died at 3 months. No medical reports could be obtained. The infant's mother had been an irregular methadone user starting 4 months prior to delivery (dose 25 to 40 mg.). A urine sample taken 6 days after treatment showed traces of quinine (evidence of heroin use). As much as 30 mg. a day of heroin was taken by the mother for 2 years preceding her pregnancy. One month after delivery, the methadone program lost contact with the mother.

Case 2

This baby died at the age of 7 1/2 weeks. The only abnormal finding was marked pulmonary congestion. The mother had used heroin for 2 years (largest daily dose about 100 mg.) and joined the methadone program one month prior to delivery. She continued taking methadone for 4 months after delivery; her urine showed no evidence of other drug use.

Case 3

This infant died at 6 1/2 weeks, in a well nourished condition. Autopsy revealed pulmonary congestion. Toxicological studies showed no evidence of drugs in the infant's blood or liver. The mother had used heroin for 1 year (largest daily use 20 mg.) and joined the methadone program seven months prior to delivery. Her daily dose was 70 mg. for the month prior to delivery. Baby was jittery at 3 hours of age with vomiting and diarrhea; he was placed on chlorpromazine for 21 days. After delivery the mother remained on methadone with no evidence of other drug use.

CONCLUSIONS

The overall expected incidence of the "sudden infant death syndrome" is about 2.5/1,000 live births. Although these deaths could be due to a chance distribution, the authors point out that methadone may be related. They rule out infant neglect as a cause of death since other infants born to heroin-using mothers are surviving in similar conditions of environmental stress. It is possible that methadone taken during pregnancy could cause some detrimental physiological or immunological change in the infant.

Rajegowda, B. K., et al. Methadone withdrawal in newborn infants.
Journal of Pediatric Research, 81(3):532-534, September 1972.

DRUG	Methadone; Heroin
SAMPLE SIZE	53
SAMPLE TYPE	Treatment (inpatient)
AGE	Neonates
SEX	Not Specified
ETHNICITY	Not Specified
GEOGRAPHICAL AREA	New York, New York
METHODOLOGY	Case Studies
DATA COLLECTION INSTRUMENT	Laboratory/Examination; Program/Clinic Statistics
DATE(S) CONDUCTED	September 1971-February 1972
NO. OF REFERENCES	4

SUMMARY

Withdrawal symptoms in a group of newborn infants of mothers on
methadone maintenance therapy were compared with those of infants
whose mothers were untreated heroin addicts.

Both the incidence and the duration of irritability and tremulousness
were greater in the methadone group than in the heroin group.

METHODOLOGY

Observations were made of 53 newborns admitted to Harlem Hospital Center between September 1971 and February 1972. Case studies compared 38 newborns of mothers addicted to heroin to 15 newborns whose mothers were on methadone maintenance.

Severity of withdrawal symptoms were noted daily by 2 authors jointly and by the nursing staff. Severity of tremors and irritability were measured by the grading system of Kahn and Associates.

Symptoms were considered present when classified as grade II (marked when the infant was disturbed) and grade III (marked at frequent intervals even when the infant was undisturbed).

Time of onset and duration of symptoms were recorded in all symptomatic methadone infants and the last 10 consecutive symptomatic heroin infants.

FINDINGS

Median birth weight among the heroin group was 2,630 grams; in the methadone group, 2,580 grams. For both groups the median gestational age was 40 weeks with a range of 34 to 40 weeks. The median 1 and 5 minute Apgar scores were similar for both groups. All 53 survived the neonatal period and none developed respiratory distress syndrome. Within the methadone group, 2 recovered from meconium aspiration and 3 full-term infants had hypoglycemia.

Only 15 out of 38 infants in the heroin addicted group went through withdrawal (mothers' "habits" varied from 2 to 30 bags daily--each bag containing approximately 19 mg of heroin).

In the methadone group, 13 out of 15 neonates suffered withdrawal symptoms (mothers' dose was 80 to 160 mg daily).

The time of onset of these symptoms in the 2 groups was comparable. Irritability lasted for a median of 7 days in the methadone group and a median of 3 days in the heroin group.

Phenobarbital sedation was required for 6 days in the methadone group and 4 days in the heroin group.

CONCLUSIONS

Methadone in the dosage utilized is addictive to the fetus. The time of onset of withdrawal symptoms is about the same for neonates born to mothers on methadone as for those born to mothers on heroin. But the incidence and duration of withdrawal symptoms is greater among neonates whose mothers are taking methadone than among neonates whose mothers are addicted to heroin.

It is the opinion of the authors that this may be a reflection of the wide range of heroin consumption, differences in properties of the two drugs, or due to a greater placental passage and/or delayed renal excretion of methadone.

More studies must be done before a final judgment can be made about the effects of methadone withdrawal on newborn infants.

Wallach, Robert C.; Jerez, Eulogio; and Blinick, George.
Pregnancy and menstrual function in narcotics addicts treated with
methadone. American Journal of Obstetrics and Gynecology,
105(8):1226-1229, December 5, 1969.

DRUG	Methadone
SAMPLE SIZE	90
SAMPLE TYPE	Treatment
AGE	Adults
SEX	Female
ETHNICITY	Not Specified
GEOGRAPHICAL AREA	New York City
METHODOLOGY	Longitudinal
DATA COLLECTION INSTRUMENT	Laboratory/Examination, Program/Clinic Statistics
DATE(S) CONDUCTED	Not Specified
NO. OF REFERENCES	20

SUMMARY

Chronic opiate addiction has been associated with amenorrhea,
anovulation, and infertility. At the Bernstein Institute of the Beth
Israel Medical Center, methadone, a synthetic narcotic, was given
daily to 95 addicted women who formerly used heroin. Twelve
women were in the menopause or had had a hysterectomy. Of the
remaining 83 premenopausal women, all but 1 resumed regular
menstruation. Thirteen pregnancies were seen, of which 8 were
conceived on high levels of methadone, and in 5 methadone therapy
was started after previous heroin addiction. All the pregnant

women were maintained on methadone, and no effect of the drug on the pregnancies has been demonstrated.

METHODOLOGY

Subjects for this test were taken from a population of 121 women who were admitted to a Methadone Maintenance Treatment Program (MMTP) over a period of 2 years. The patients were all hard-core "mainliners," intravenous heroin addicts, with histories of numerous arrests, multiple drug exposures, and repeated experiences with the detoxification program.

Care was taken in selecting patients for the MMTP to avoid street addicts with multiple drug abuse, alcoholism, and schizophrenia. Patients were given increasingly larger dosages until a daily morning dose of 60 to 120 mg. was received by 13 subjects prior to, during, and following pregnancy. In 5 patients methadone maintenance treatment was begun during pregnancy.

Of the 121 women originally admitted to the program, a total of 90 were of reproductive age at the time of the study. Seven of the 90 had hysterectomies; one while under treatment. Five were postmenopausal. Eleven of the 12 fathers of the recorded pregnancies were participating in the same treatment program.

FINDINGS

While on heroin prior to entering the program, 67% stated that they menstruated infrequently or not at all; 19% stated that their menses were normal. While on methadone maintenance, 82 women began to menstruate regularly, usually within 1 to 2 months. Thirteen pregnancies were recorded in women ranging in age from 24 to 36 years. All but 1 had had 1 or more pregnancies before entering the program. The interval since their prior pregnancies varied from 2 to 9 years.

The antepartum course on all pregnancies was uneventful with no toxemia or undue weight gain. One patient with a possible serology was treated with penicillin. Of the 13 pregnancies, 2 were undelivered at the time of reporting. There were 8 live deliveries, 7 by the vaginal route and one by repeat caesarean section. There was a stillborn vaginal delivery with death due to umbilical cord strangulation, 2 spontaneous or induced abortions, and one ectopic pregnancy.

CONCLUSIONS

Ovulation, conception and pregnancy seemed to have been little affected by significant dosages of methadone; the abortion rate could not be evaluated in such a small series. High average maternal age was consistent with the higher ages seen in women in the detoxification program. The uniform return to a regular menstrual pattern in all but 1 of the 83 patients of menstrual age was considered a striking finding and was attributed to the concurrent return to an orderly existence or a pharmacologic effect of the methadone, which may differ from heroin. The MMTP program stabilized the life of the addict by largely removing the usual stresses and malnutrition, and the patients were kept under constant medical surveillance.

V. METHADONE AND HEROIN: COMPARATIVE STUDIES

Rementeria, Jose Luis, and Nunag, Nemesio N. Narcotic withdrawal in pregnancy: Stillbirth incidence with a case report. American Journal of Obstetrics and Gynecology, 116 (8): 1152-1156, August 15, 1973.

DRUG	Methadone and Heroin
SAMPLE SIZE	47
SAMPLE TYPE	Treatment (inpatient)
AGE	Neonatal
SEX	Both Male and Female
ETHNICITY	Not Specified
GEOGRAPHICAL AREA	Bronx, New York
METHODOLOGY	Case Study
DATA COLLECTION INSTRUMENT	Observations, Laboratory/Examination, and Program/Clinic Statistics
DATE(S) CONDUCTED	January 15, 1971 to July 15, 1972
NO. OF REFERENCES	22

SUMMARY

The authors studied infants born to narcotic-addicted mothers and found that the stillbirth rate among them was 4 times that of the general obstetric population.

In this paper one case study is presented in an attempt to analyze the particulars of stillbirth associated with narcotic withdrawal in pregnancy.

CASE STUDY

A 23-year-old pregnant heroin addict began withdrawal symptoms during her 39th week of pregnancy. Labor contractions followed shortly. The woman took another injection of heroin and went to the hospital. The admitting physician could not detect fetal heart sounds even though the mother had felt fetal movement upon arrival at the hospital. Labor continued. Several hours later the woman delivered (vaginally) a stillborn female infant. Post mortem examination of the infant revealed large quantities of meconium in the amniotic fluid, the infant's mouth, nose, trachea, bronchi and lungs. In addition there were focal hemorrhages and congestion in the visceral organs, spleen, kidney, ovaries, liver and adrenal glands.

COMMENTS

When a pregnant addict goes into withdrawal, it is believed that the fetus does likewise. Under this stress, two things happen: the fetus passes meconium and initiates strong respiratory movements. If withdrawal coincides with labor, death could occur due to the following factors:

(1)   Withdrawal increases muscular activity, which increases the already high metabolic rate and oxygen consumption level of the fetus.

(2)   The older the fetus, the higher its metabolic rate.

(3)   During labor with contractions compromising the blood flow through the uterus and thus effecting oxygen circulation, such an increased need for oxygen might not be met.

(4)   If the fetus were exposed to insufficient oxygen for any length of time, hypoxia and/or death might occur.

CONCLUSIONS

The authors' study, carried out over 18 months at Fordham Hospital, illustrates in two tables a higher incidence of stillborn and neonatal deaths among heroin-addicted mothers than most previous studies showed. This difference is attributed to the low number of methadone maintenance pregnancies in this particular study as compared to the others. The chances of a pregnant addict being able to get enough heroin to prevent withdrawal, as in the case study, are low in contrast to the steady maintenance fo methadone. Thus, the rate of fetal and neonatal deaths would be higher.

When withdrawal and labor coincide, hypoxia and death may follow, since one effect of withdrawal is to increase the need for oxygen over and above what may be supplied during labor. But the effects of withdrawal on the fetus during pregnancy need further clarification in certain areas, and studies need to be done of infants who have survived severe intrauterine withdrawal. The authors do not attempt to explain the mechanism of intrauterine anoxia. It is recommended that addicts be "maintained" rather than "withdrawn" during pregnancy.

Finnegan, Loretta P.; Connaughton, James F.; Emich, John P.; et al. Comprehensive care of the pregnant addict and its effect on maternal and infant outcome. Contemporary Drug Problems, 1(4):795-809, Fall 1972.

DRUG	Heroin
SAMPLE SIZE	85
SAMPLE TYPE	Treatment: inpatient and outpatient
AGE	Group A, average 26; Group B, 24 years
SEX	Female
ETHNICITY	Not Specified
GEOGRAPHICAL AREA	Philadelphia
METHODOLOGY	Controlled/Experimental
DATA COLLECTION INSTRUMENT	Interview, Clinical Tests.
DATE(S) CONDUCTED	Jan. 1969-Aug. 1970, Sept. 1970-Dec. 1971
NO. OF REFERENCES	10

SUMMARY

This study explored the increasing health problem of pregnant narcotic addicts. It investigated two groups of women admitted to the Philadelphia General Hospital between 1969-1971--Group A receiving no prenatal care, Group B being enrolled in the special prenatal clinic in a methadone maintenance program. It was found that treated patients (Group B) experienced fewer obstetrical complications.

METHODOLOGY

In an attempt to discover and reduce obstetrical and medical problems of drug-addicted pregnant women a comprehensive treatment program was developed at the Philadelphia General Hospital. This program was designed to permit evaluation of the morbidity and mortality of the pregnant addict and her child. A special prenatal clinic was established in September, 1970, and the patients examined there were known narcotic addicts. At their initial prenatal visit, a history was obtained and a physical examination performed. The patient was subsequently given a chest film, a urinalysis, blood tests, including C.B.C., Serology, Bloodtype, and an SMA-12. Initial prenatal counseling was given, including an abortion option in early pregnancy. Discussions were held regarding the relationship of heroin addiction to the serious complications of pregnancy, and if the patient was not already receiving therapy for her addiction, she was referred to the F.D.A. approved methadone program at the hospital.

Subsequently, counseling was given on withdrawal problems, nutrition, fetal and maternal changes, the process of labor, delivery, and anesthesia. After delivery the mother was admitted to the obstetrical intensive care unit and maintained on methadone with subsequent referral to the methadone clinic upon discharge.

Two groups of addicts were studied at the hospital: <u>Group A</u>. Pregnant narcotic addicts who delivered at Philadelphia General Hospital from January, 1969 through August, 1970, the period before the comprehensive care program began. In addition, addicts (street addicts on heroin) who delivered at the hospital from September, 1970, through December, 1971, who had no prenatal care and no methadone, were also included in this control group. There were 29 patients in this group. <u>Group B</u>. Pregnant narcotic patients who were enrolled in the special prenatal clinic and in the methadone maintenance program who delivered infants between September, 1970, and December, 1971. There were 56 patients in this group.

FINDINGS

Medical complications occurred in 41% of the control group (A) and in 24% of the treated group (B). The complications seen in both groups were anemia, syphilis, serum hepatitis, hypertension, kidney disease, and cellulitis. In the untreated group, anemia, serum hepatitis, kidney disease, and cellulitis occurred with greater frequency, whereas syphilis and hypertension alone, without toxemia, occurred more often in the treated group. In the control group 52% of the 29 patients manifested one or more obstetrical complications,whereas in the treated group, 24% of the 56 patients had complications. Pre-eclampsia was diagnosed in 15% of the control patients and in 5% of the treated patients. Premature rupture of membranes, of 24 hours duration or more, was found in 15% of the control patients and in 9% of the treated patients. 3% of control patients developed amnionitis, but none of the treated group did. Fetal distress occurred during labor in 15% of the control group and in 7% of the treated group. Post partum hemorrhage did not occur in the treated group, but 7% of the control patients manifested this complication.

After birth the infant was admitted to the Neonatal Intensive Care Unit for careful observation of symptoms of withdrawal. When they occurred, close observation continued until progression of symptoms was noted and then therapy was promptly instituted. It was found that 50%-75% of infants born to heroin addicts will manifest symptoms of withdrawal. The incidence of low birth weight in Group A was 48%, and in Group B it was 24%. The average weight of infants born to the control patients (A) was 2485 grams, and in the treated patients (B), it was 2600 grams.

CONCLUSIONS

The study of the untreated group correlates with other reports in the literature. In the treated group of patients, however, a reduction in the incidence of toxemia has been achieved, lower than that regularly reported at the Philadelphia General Hospital. The usual figure was 8%. Therefore, it appears advantageous to instigate special programs for treating pregnant addicts.

Zelson, Carl; Lee, Sook Ja; and Casalino, Marie. Neonatal narcotic addiction: Comparative effects of maternal intake of heroin and methadone. The New England Journal of Medicine, 289(23): 1216-1220, December 6, 1973.

DRUG	Methadone and Heroin
SAMPLE SIZE	91
SAMPLE TYPE	Treatment (inpatient)
AGE	91 Neonates
SEX	Not Specified
ETHNICITY	Not Specified
GEOGRAPHICAL AREA	New York City
METHODOLOGY	Exploratory/Descriptive
DATA COLLECTION INSTRUMENT	Observations, Laboratory/Examination
DATE(S) CONDUCTED	July 1971 to December 31, 1972.
NO. OF REFERENCES	14

SUMMARY

From July 1, 1971, to December 31, 1972, 91 infants born at Metropolitan Hospital in New York City were children of drug-addicted mothers. Forty-six of the mothers were methadone addicts, and 45 were heroin addicts.

Because of an increase in use of methadone by pregnant addicts, this study concerned itself with the effects of methadone and heroin on their infants.

In comparing the infants, it was found that withdrawal syndrome occurred with equal frequency in both groups, but signs of withdrawal and severity of such signs were greater among methadone-exposed infants.

METHODOLOGY

Infants of 46 methadone-addicted mothers were compared to infants of 45 heroin-addicted mothers. All the infants were observed for signs of withdrawal. The study was undertaken for an 18-month period from July 7, 1971, to December 31, 1972. The infants were studied at Metropolitan Hospital, New York City.

FINDINGS

Seventy-six percent of the heroin infants and 91% of the methadone infants showed signs of withdrawal. There was no statistically significant difference between the two groups. Onset of withdrawal signs occurred for most of the infants within the first 48 hours of life. Tremors, hypertonicity, irritability, vomiting and respiratory distress were the most frequent signs noted. It was quite apparent that the methadone babies had more withdrawal signs than the heroin babies.

There were infants of mothers who had been on both methadone and heroin in unspecified quantities during their pregnancies. This group also showed more frequent and severe signs of withdrawal than the heroin group.

Infants with 3 or more withdrawal signs that became more severe were treated with chlorpromazine.

This study demonstrated that ingestion of methadone during pregnancy, whether taken for short periods or for the entire pregnancy, would affect the unborn child. Infants whose mothers used methadone had a more severe withdrawal syndrome than is usually seen in infants born to heroin-addicted mothers. The mean age of the methadone mothers was 22.8, and that of the heroin mothers 20.5. Forty-seven percent of the heroin-addicted and 42% of the methadone addicted mothers attended a prenatal clinic. Low-birth-weight infants in these groups may have been the result of intrauterine exposure to the maternal narcotic intake.

The data presented in this study demonstrated that infants born to addicted mothers are more severely affected by the intrauterine exposure to methadone than to heroin; whether these effects are temporary or of a prolonged nature may only be determined by a long follow-up period.

CONCLUSIONS

The results of this study indicated a marked difference in the infants of methadone-addicted mothers, as opposed to infants of heroin-addicted mothers. The authors feel that switching pregnant addicts from heroin to methadone can bring about consequences detrimental to the newborn. It is their opinion that methadone should not be used indiscriminately during pregnancy.

Reddy, A. Mahender; Harper, Rita G.; and Stern, Gertrude. Observations on heroin and methadone withdrawal in the newborn.
Pediatrics, 48(3): 353-357, September, 1971.

DRUG	Heroin
SAMPLE SIZE	45
SAMPLE TYPE	Treatment (inpatient)
AGE	Neonates
SEX	19 Male, 21 Female
ETHNICITY	37 Black, 1 Puerto Rican, 2 White
GEOGRAPHICAL AREA	New York
METHODOLOGY	Case Studies
DATA COLLECTION INSTRUMENT	Observations
DATE(S) CONDUCTED	1967-1970
NO. OF REFERENCES	13

SUMMARY

Retrospective analysis of 40 infants born to heroin addicts showed
that 85% developed withdrawal symptoms: central nervous system,
gastrointestinal and respiratory disturbances. At delivery, respiratory depression was not a prominent feature. This suggests that
tolerance to chronic narcotic usage develops even in utero.

The study substantiates a high incidence of low birth weight infants,
previously noted by other studies. Over 50% of the infants were

small for gestational age, rather than true premature infants. Morbidity was high, but only 2 infants, both below 1,000 gm. birth weight, died. Serious congenital malformations were not observed. Withdrawal symptoms were also noted in infants born to methadone-maintained mothers. They showed similar withdrawal patterns to those from heroin-addicted mothers. The authors suggest that pediatricians should be aware that such infants may be seriously compromised in the newborn period.

METHODOLOGY

The study analyzed retrospectively the course of 40 infants born to admitted heroin users between July, 1967, and June, 1970. Maternal age ranged from 16 to 35, 77% being between 20 and 25. Racial distribution (37 Black, 2 White, 1 Puerto Rican) reflected the hospital population; 19 were male, 21 female. All infants were observed from birth until they were discharged in good condition, or had died. Thirty-one infants were treated for withdrawal symptoms with either paregoric therapy or phenobarbital.

FINDINGS

Examination revealed that 25 were below 2,500 gm. at birth. Seven were true premature infants, 18 were small for gestational age, and 15 were full term. Apgar scores ranged between 3 and 9. Almost all were in good condition at delivery, with 31 of the infants receiving an Apgar score of 5 or above. No infants revealed serious congenital malformations.

Six infants (15%) were asymptomatic, while 34 (85%) showed withdrawal symptoms consisting primarily of disturbances of the central nervous system, as well as respiratory or gastrointestinal problems. Twenty-three exhibited these symptoms prior to 24 hours of age. Hyperactivity, irritability, and tremors were also observed, and, less frequently, high temperatures, nasal congestion, and tachypnea. Forty-four manifested poor feeding, vomiting or diarrhea, usually between the 4th and 6th day. Blood sugar and blood calcium were normal, as were hematocrit levels.

Withdrawal symptoms of varying severity lasted an average of 4 days, and were treated with paregoric (23 subjects) or phenobarbital (8 subjects). The latter required shorter treatment (18 days) than the former (1 month).

Observations of 5 other infants whose mothers were receiving methadone, revealed that these infants manifested withdrawal symptoms of tremors, irritability, excessive crying, hyperactivity, hyperthermia, and gastrointestinal disturbances.

CONCLUSIONS

Early onset of symptoms requires that infants born to heroin-addicted mothers be identified before delivery and closely observed during the perinatal period.

The etiology of the symptoms of infants born to methadone-maintained mothers is unclear. Two interpretations are suggested. Either methadone produces a withdrawal pattern similar to heroin, or the mothers may have used heroin in addition to methadone. Further study is suggested.

The authors were surprised at the lack of low Apgar scores. This suggests tolerance to narcotic usage even in utero.

High incidence of low birth weight leads the authors to suggest considering the growth-retarding effects of heroin, or of quinine with which heroin is often cut. The study does not support the concept of a high incidence of serious congenital malformations or high mortality.

VI.   SELECTED ANNOTATED STUDIES

Finnegan, Loretta P.; Connaughton, James F.; and Emich, John P.
Abstinence score in the treatment of the infant of the drug-
dependent mother. Pediatric Research, 7(4): 319/91, April 1973.

SUMMARY

Over the past 3 years, 85% of 146 infants of drug-dependent mothers
at P.G.H. manifested symptoms of abstinence. In the management
of the first 121 infants careful observation for the onset and progression of symptoms preceded the use of drugs in the therapeutic regimen.
Thus far the decision to use drugs or to increase dosage was influenced by arbitrarily applied clinical criteria providing inadequate
basis for judgement in the treatment of this syndrome. A neonatal
abstinence score has been devised to provide a more precise method
of management in the last 25 infants of drug-dependent mothers.
Twenty-one of the commonly seen symptoms are listed and each has
been given a score of 1-5 according to its clinical significance (i.e.,
convulsion = 5, sweating = 1). The infants are scored once every hour
for the first 24 hrs., every 2 hrs. for the second 24 hrs., and every
4 hrs. for the duration of symptomatology. Infants whose score is 7
or less are not treated with drugs. Once a score of 8 or more is
attained and sustained for 3 hrs., the infant is treated. Dosage
schedules relating the score to particular dosages of detoxicant drugs
are used. (The higher the score the greater the mg/kg/day of drug.)
This abstinence score will be helpful in monitoring the symptomatology
of the passively addicted infant and may provide more uniform criteria
for assessment and treatment.

Glass, Leonard, and Evans, Hugh E. Narcotic withdrawal in the
    newborn. American Family Physician, 6(1):75-78, July, 1972.

SUMMARY

The two most commonly employed narcotic drugs are heroin and
methadone. Most pregnant addicts have a history of very poor
diets and little or no obstetric care; in addition their general health
is suboptimal. The increasing availability of methadone programs to
pregnant addicts has increased the number of those seeking prenatal
care. Over 50 percent of the infants born to narcotic addicted mothers
are of low birth weight (less than 2,500 gms.); half of these are premature by date, with a gestational age of less than 38 weeks. There is
a high incidence of complications, such as fetal anoxia with aspiration
of meconium. The respiratory distress syndrome is rarely encountered,
even in infants whose gestational age places them at highest risk.
Symptoms of narcotic withdrawal usually begin during the first day of
life and infrequently first appear on the second or third day. Infants of
mothers who are on methadone maintenance with doses over 100 mg. /
day usually show symptoms of withdrawal. The immediate prognosis
for addicted infants is generally good; recovery is usually complete by
the end of their first week of life. Deaths are unusual and are
associated with a medical complication, such as prematurity or
infection.

Glass, Leonard, et.al. Effect of heroin on cortisol production
in pregnant addicts and their fetuses. Pediatric Research, 7(4):
320/92, April, 1973.

SUMMARY

In order to assess the effects of heroin (which freely crosses the
placenta) on fetal and maternal adrenocortical function, cord sera
cortisol concentrations were determined by a fluorometric assay
method (BMJ 2:310, 1972) on 18 non-asphyxiated infants of addicted
mothers and 15 infants of nonaddicted mothers of similar birth weights
and gestational ages. All infants were born by normal vaginal delivery. Cortisol levels were also determined in blood of 17 addicted
and 12 nonaddicted mothers, drawn at the time of delivery.

While serum cortisol levels were comparable in both study (median
12. 3 mg/100ml; range 8. 3-20. 6 mg/100ml) and control (median 13. 0;
range 4. 8-21. 0 mg/100ml) infants, addicted mothers had significantly
lower concentrations (median 22. 7 mg/100ml; range 12. 0-71. 0 mg./
100ml) than nonaddicted mothers (median 38. 5 mg/100ml; range 23. 8-
75. 5 mg/100ml) (p<0. 01).

Heroin decreases cortisol production in adults by inhibiting secretion
of ACTH. Decreased levels were found in pregnant addicts at the time
of delivery; however, values were similar in infants of addicted and
nonaddicted mothers. The reason for these differences has not been
explained. The findings may reflect a decreased responsiveness of
the fetal pituitary to heroin or a relative insensitivity of the fetal
adrenal cortex to fluctuations in ACTH secretion.

Kandall, Stephen R.; and Gartner, Lawrence M. Delayed presentation of neonatal methadone withdrawal. <u>Pediatric Research</u>,
7(4): 320/92, April 1973.

SUMMARY

Infants born of mothers with methadone addiction have been recognized
recently to have more severe and prolonged symptoms of withdrawal
than do infants born to mothers with heroin addiction. It has not been
previously recognized, however, that methadone addicted infants may
also have onset of initial symptoms of withdrawal late in the newborn
period following an initial period of 2 to 4 weeks without symptoms.
Of 71 infants at the Bronx Municipal Hospital Center in 1972 developing symptoms of narcotic withdrawal, 46 were born of mothers
using methadone alone or in combination with heroin. Five of these
46 methadone addicted infants developed their initial symptoms between 2 and 4 weeks of age. Symptoms at presentation were similar
to those observed in infants with early onset, but in one case the
initial symptoms were seizures and in another the infant died at home
following symptoms of increasing irritablity and diarrhea.

The markedly increased usage of methadone and its severe and prolonged withdrawal symptoms in the newborn, coupled with the recognition that these symptoms may be silent for 2 to 4 weeks after birth,
makes this a major public health problem. Further study of the developmental pharmacology of methadone in the neonate is needed, and
increased surveillance of such potentially addicted infants is
mandatory.

Kron, Reuben E. ; Litt, Mitchell; and Finnegan, Loretta P.
  Behavior of infants born to narcotic-addicted mothers.
  Pediatric Research, 7(4):292/64, April 1973.

SUMMARY

This report describes abnormalities in the nutritive sucking performance of congenitally addicted infants undergoing narcotic
withdrawal.

A series of 50 infants born to mothers addicted either to heroin or to
methadone were studied by an objective method for measuring sucking
behavior. Sucking rates as well as average pressures and amounts of
nutrient consumed during sucking were significantly reduced for the
addicted infants relative to a control group born to normal mothers
and a second control group born to toxemic mothers. The subgroup
of infants born to methadone-addicted mothers was significantly more
depressed with regard to sucking behavior than the infants of heroin-
addicted mothers. Furthermore infants treated with paregoric (an
opiate) for symptoms of the narcotic withdrawal syndrome showed
significantly less depression of the sucking response than those treated
with sedatives such as phenobarbital. These results raise questions
about a number of a priori assumptions regarding the safety and
efficacy of current treatment methods for maternal and neonatal
addiction.

Lipsitz, Philip J.; and Blatman, Saul. The early neonatal period of 100 live-borns of mothers on methadone. Pediatric Research, 7(4):404/176, April 1973.

SUMMARY

From January 1967 to January 1973, we have taken care of 100 new-borns delivered to mothers taking methadone. The dose of methadone taken was from 40 to 120 mg. daily. Only 5 pregnant patients were on doses of 50 mg. or less. All the newborns at delivery had Apgar scores greater than 6 and the majority scored more than 7 at one minute. The mean birthweight was 2,786 grams (range 1,176 to 4,338 grams). Gestational age was 30 to 40 weeks. Twenty-six weighed 2,500 grams or less and of these 54% were A.G.A. and 46% S.G.A. The sex ratio was male: female 1.2:1. A major congenital anomaly was noted in 1 newborn and 2 had supernumerary digits. There were 2 neonatal deaths in this group. Symptomatology of narcotic withdrawal was graded according to the system of Kahn, et al., (Journal of Pediatrics, 75:495, 1969). Grade II symptoms occurred in 53% and grade III in 5%. Three newborns had seizure-like activity. We propose a numerical scoring value of withdrawal symptoms so that everyone dealing with these newborns uses a standard grading system. The onset of symptoms occurred in the first 4 days of life in 78% of the symptomatic newborn. Bilirubin levels > 13 mg% occurred in 14%. The newborns were observed in the hospital for a mean of 16 days (range 7-78). All but 8 were discharged in care of the mother.

Naeye, Richard L.; Blanc, William A.; and Leblanc, Werner.
Heroin and the fetus. <u>Pediatric Research</u>, 7(4):321/93, April, 1973.

SUMMARY

Many neonates of mothers on heroin have small birth weights. Both
fetal growth retardation and preterm delivery are at fault. Autopsy
material was examined from: (a) 29 newborns whose mothers used
heroin only up to delivery; (b) 10 neonates whose mothers used heroin
only in early pregnancy; (c) 3 infants with mothers on methadone;
(d) 7 neonates whose nonaddicted mothers had hepatitis; (e) 1,044
newborn controls; (f) placentas from 28 surviving infants of heroin
addicts. The percent preterm (<38 weeks) infants in the group was:
(a) 83%; (b) 50%; (c) 100%; (d) 86%; (e) 78%. The incidence of the
amniotic fluid infection syndrome: (a) 57%; (b) 70%; (c) 0%; (d) 27%;
(e) 54%. The incidence of hyaline membrane disease in the infants:
(a) 40%; (b) 0%; (c) 67%; (d) 57%. Body weights in percentages of
normal values: (a) 86%; (b) 99%; (c) 114%; (d) 103%; (e) 106%. Using
quantitative methods, the subnormal size of organs in neonates of
heroin addicts was due to a subnormal number of cells at all gestational
ages. Near term infants had cells with a subnormal cytoplasmic
mass. All the organ abnormalities can be explained by differing
effects of maternal undernutrition at the various gestational ages.
The amniotic infection syndrome appears responsible for many pre-
term deliveries.

Naeye, Richard L.; Blanc, William; and LeBlanc, Werner. Postmortem findings in offspring of heroin addicts, Laboratory
Investigation, 28(3):392-393, 1973.

ABSTRACT

Offspring of heroin addicts are reported to have an excessive rate of
prematurity and perinatal mortality but a low incidence of the respiratory distress syndrome whose most common cause is hyaline
membrane disease. We analyzed autopsy material from (a) 29 newborns whose mothers used heroin up to delivery, (b) 10 newborns
whose mothers used heroin only during early pregnancy, (c) 3 newborns whose mothers were on methadone, (d) 1044 newborn controls,
and (e) placentas from 28 surviving offspring of heroin addicts. The
incidence of hyaline membrane disease in "at risk" infants of the
various groups was: (a) 40 percent, (b) 0 percent, (c) 67 percent,
(d) 57 percent. The incidence of the amniotic fluid infection syndrome
with congenital pneumonia was (a) 57 percent, (b) 70 percent, (c) 0
percent, (d) 27 percent, (e) 54 percent (placentitis). Other abnormalities in groups a and b were: intraventricular hemorrhage, four
cases; subarachnoid hemorrhage, four cases; pulmonary hemorrhage,
two cases; pneumothorax, one case; congenital cardiac malformation,
one case. Thus, no specific disease process or fetal abnormality can
be directly related to heroin, but the excessive prematurity and perinatal deaths in offspring of addicts appear related to the amniotic fluid
infection syndrome.

Zelson, C.; and Lee, S.J. Neonatal narcotic addiction-exposure to heroin and methadone. <u>Pediatric Research</u>, 7(4):289/61, April 1973.

<u>SUMMARY</u>

Over the past 12 years, we have cared for more than 550 infants born to heroin addicted mothers. Approximately one-half of the infants required treatment. Recently, we have observed many gravidae on methadone alone or in combination with heroin. Their addicted infants appear to be more ill than those born to mothers on heroin. 12% of infants born of mothers on heroin required treatment, while 38% born to mothers on methadone were treated. Over a recent 13-month period, 58 infants were observed, 34 born to mothers who had used methadone alone or in combination with heroin, and 24 to mothers only on heroin. A comparison of the 2 groups showed the following: 1. the incidence of low-birth-weight infants was similar; 2. among infants born to mothers on methadone, weight and gestational age were more frequently concordant than for infants born to heroin addicted mothers; 3. methadone infants have higher average birth weights; 4. Apgar scores were lower in infants exposed to methadone; 5. the severity of withdrawal and the number of signs in each instance were greater in methadone infants; 6. seizures were also more frequent in methadone infants; 8. hyaline membrane disease occurred in methadone infants, but has not been seen in heroin infants.

SELECTIVE BIBLIOGRAPHY

Annunziato, D. Neonatal addiction to methadone. Pediatrics, 47:787, April, 1971.

Baker, J.B.E. The effects of drugs on the foetus. Pharmacological Reviews, 12(1):37-41, 81-90, 1960.

Connaughton, J.F.; Finnegan, L.; Wieland, W.Q.; and Polin, J.I. Current concepts in management of pregnant narcotic addicts. Obstetrics and Gynecology, 37(4):631, 1971.

Gaulden, E.C.; Littlefield, D.C.; Putoff, O.E.; and Seivert, A.L. Menstrual abnormalities associated with heroin addiction. American Journal of Obstetrics and Gynecology, 90:155-160, 1964.

Hall, R.J. Teratogenic and Chromosomal Damaging Effects of Illicit Drugs. An Annotated Bibliography. Toronto, Ontario, Canada: Addiction Research Foundation, 1973.

Hoey, J. LSD and chromosome damage. Journal of the American Medical Association, 212:1707, June 8, 1970.

Lynch, H.T., and Kaplan, A.R. Genetic counseling and drugs. Paediatrician, 1:26-34, 1972.

Moorhead, P.S.; Jarvik, L.F.; and Cohen, M.M. Cytogenetic methods for mutagenicity testing. In: Epstein, Samuel S., ed. Drugs of Abuse. Their Genetic and Other Chronic Nonpsychiatric Hazards. Cambridge, Masschusetts: Massachusetts Institute of Technology Press, 1971. pp. 140-170.

Naeye, R.L., and Blanc, W. Fetal growth in offspring of heroin addicts. A quantitive study. American Journal of Pathology, 70(2):85a, February, 1973.

Nathenson, G.; Cohen M.I.; Litt, I.F.; and McNamara, H. The effect of maternal heroin addiction on neonatal jaundice. Journal of Pediatrics, 81(5):899-903, 1972.

Nichols, Warren W. Genetic hazards of drugs of abuse. In:
    Zarafonetis, Chris J.D., ed., Drug Abuse: Proceedings of the
    International Conference on Drug Abuse, Ann Arbor, Michigan,
    November 9-13, 1970. Philadelphia: Lea and Febiger, 1972.
    pp. 93-99.

Schweigert, F.B. Neonatal barbiturate withdrawal. Journal of the
    American Medical Association, 221:1282, September 11, 1972.

Zelson, C.; Kahn, E.J.; and Neumann, L. Heroin withdrawal
    syndrome. Journal of Pediatrics, 76:483-484, March, 1970.

INDEXES

The numbers in the indexes refer to the unique identification code found in the upper right-hand corner on the first page of each abstract. Roman numerals reference categories from the Table of Contents; Arabic numerals reference abstracts within categories. It should be pointed out that a given index term refers to an entire abstract rather than to pages within an abstract.

The keyword terms selected for the indexes are those terms used in the literature; no terms were inferred. The most specific term was used whenever possible. Thus, some material on marijuana will be found under that term but other material may be found under the term cannabis. Similarly, studies of heroin use may be indexed under heroin but also under opiates.

For convenience to the reader, the indexes have been divided into the following five sections:

Drugs

Includes general and specific names of all drugs mentioned in the abstract, as used by the authors of the document.

Sample Types

Terms which describe as specifically as possible the sample population studied.

Geographic Locations

Organized by state, the location where the study was carried out; includes also names of universities, schools, drug programs, committees, etc., in the order in which they occur in the abstracts.

Subjects

Terms which describe the subjects or concepts of the studies; included also are names of specific data collection instruments, evaluation tools, and questionnaires.

Authors

All authors named in the citation to each abstract are listed in the author index; however, this does not include all authors of the materials abstracted since documents with more than two authors have been cited with et al.

AUTHORS

Antopol, W.   III.08
Auld, P.   III.10
Barton, W.   III.01
Bateman, K.   II.04
Beaumont, G.   IV.02
Behrendt, H.   III.13
Berlin, C.   II.09
Blanc, W.   VI.07, VI.08
Blatman, S.   VI.06
Bleyer, W.   I.09
Blinick, G.   III.08, IV.05
Brazelton, T.   I.04
Cohen, M.   II.08
Connaughton, J.   V.02, VI.01
Conrad, D.   III.12
Crow, J.   I.02
Desmond, M.   I.08, III.14
Dumars, K.   II.05
Einstein, S.   I.01
Eller, J.   II.10
Emich, J.   V.02, VI.01
Evans, H.   III.12, VI.02
Falek, A.   I.01
Finnegan, L.   V.01, V.02,
   VI.05
Floyd, M.   III.09
Forfar, J.   I.03
Gartner, L.   VI.04
Glass, L.   III.09, III.12,
   VI.02, VI.03
Golden, G.   III.16
Green, M.   III.13
Greenblatt, D.   II.03
Harper, R.   V.04
Hill, R.   III.14
Hirschhorn, K.   II.08
Howard, P.   IV.03
Jacobson, C.   II.09
Jarvis, J.   II.07
Jerez, E.   IV.05
Kahn, E.   III.09, III.15
Kandall, S.   VI.04

Klain, D.   III.10
Kleber, H.   IV.03
Krause, S.   III.03
Krauss, A.   III.10
Kron, R.   VI.05
Leblanc, W.   VI.07, VI.08
Lee, S.   VI.09
Lin-Fu, J.   III.02
Lipsitz, P.   VI.06
Litt, I.   III.16
Litt, M.   VI.05
Long, S.   II.01
Marshall, R.   I.09
Maslansky, R.   IV.02
Morton, J.   II.10
Naeye, R.   III.11, VI.07, VI.08
Nathenson, G.   III.16
Nelson, M.   I.03
Neuberg, R.   I.07
Neumann, L.   I.06, III.15
Nunag, N.   V.01
Pierson, P.   IV.03
Polk, G.   III.15
Rajegowda, B.   III.09, III.12,
   IV.04
Reddy, A.   V.04
Rementeria, J.   V.01
Rimoin, D.   II.06
Rubio, E.   III.06
Schulman, C.   III.07
Schwanecke, R.   I.08
Shader, R.   II.03
Sly, W.   II.06
Smart, R.   II.04
Statzer, D.   IV.01
Stencherer, M.   II.07
Stern, G.   V.04
Stern, R.   III.05
Stone, M.   III.04
Sukov, R.   IV.02
Sussman, S.   I.05
Titus, R.   II.02

Wallach, R.   IV.05
Wardell, J.   IV.01
Warren, R.   II.06
Wasserman, E.   III.06
William, N.   III.08
Wilson, G.   I.08
Zelson, C.   III.06, V.03,
    VI.09

DRUGS

alcohol   I.03, I.04, I.07,
    I.09, IV.05
amphetamines   I.03, I.05,
    I.06, I.07, II.05, II.09
anesthetics   I.03, I.04, I.06
barbiturates   I.03, I.04, I.05,
    I.07, I.08, I.09, II.05,
    II.09, III.03, III.14
cannabis   I.07, II.06
chlorpromazine   I.07, II.08,
    III.04, III.14, III.15, IV.03,
    V.03
cocaine   II.05
codine   I.04, I.05
glue   II.05
hallucinogens   I.06
hashish   II.05
heroin   I.05, I.06, I.07, I.08,
    II.09, III (all), IV.01, IV.04,
    IV.05, V (all), VI.02, VI.03,
    VI.04, VI.07, VI.08, VI.09
hypnotics   I.03
LSD   I.01, I.04, I.06, IV.02,
    II (all)
marijuana   I.05, II.05, II.09
meperdine   I.04
mescaline   II.05, II.09
methadone   I.07, III.03, III.04,
    III.14, IV (all), V (all), VI.02,
    VI.04, VI.05, VI.06, VI.08,
    VI.09
methedrine   I.05, I.07
Mongolism   III.03

morphine   I.05, I.06, III.06
paregorics   V.04, VI.05
peyote   II.06, II.09
phenobarbital   I.05, I.07, I.08,
    I.09, III.09, III.14, III.15,
    IV.01, IV.04, V.04, VI.05
polycystic kidneys   III.03
progesterone   I.04
promethazine   I.05
quinine   III.06, IV.01, IV.03,
    V.04
severe tolipes equinovarus   III.03
STP   II.05, II.09
subtentorial hematoma   III.03
subdural hemorrhage   III.03
Tincture of Opium   IV.01
tobacco   I.03, I.09, II.09, II.10,
    III.13
tranquilizers   I.03, I.04, I.06,
    II.05, III.04
Valium   III.16

STUDY TYPES

animal studies   II.01, II.04
chromosome evaluation I.01,
    II (all)
dominant lethal assays   I.01
Drosophila   I.01
epidemiological surveillance   I.02,
    I.03
in vitro   I.01, II.01, II.02, II.03,
    II.04, II.07, II.08
in vivo   I.01, I.02, II.01, II.02,
    II.06, II.07, II.08
microbial studies   I.01, I.02
phenotypic abnormalities   I.02
somatic cytogenetic   I.02

GEOGRAPHIC LOCATOR

California   I.05, II.05
Colorado   II.10
Connecticut   IV.03
District of Columbia   II.09, III.01

Kentucky   III.02
Michigan   IV.01
Minnesota   IV.02
Missouri   II.05
New York   III.02, III.03,
    III.04, III.05, III.06, III.07,
    III.08, III.09, III.10, III.11,
    III.02, III.13, III.15, III.16,
    IV.04, V.01, V.03, V.04,
    VI.04
Ohio   II.07
Pennsylvania   V.02
Texas   I.08, III.14
Washington   I.09

Scotland, Edinburgh   I.03

SUBJECTS

abortions   I.07, II.06, II.08,
    II.09, III.02
abruptio placenta   III.02
abscesses   I.06
acid-base status   III.09,
    III.10
anemia   V.02
Apgar scores   I.08, I.09, IV.04,
    V.04, VI.06
banding techniques   I.01
breech births   I.05, I.06, II.09,
    III.02, III.04, III.05
cellulitis   I.05
congenital defects   I.01, I.02,
    II.06, II.08, II.10, III.06,
    IV.02, VI.06
convulsions   I.05, I.06, I.07
EEG's   I.04, I.09, III.07
EKG   I.09, III.07
EMG   III.07
endocarditis   I.06
epileptic   mothers   I.08
genetics   I.01
hepatitis   I.05, I.06, III.02,
    III.04, III.11

hypoglycemia   IV.04
irritability   I.09, III.02, III.12,
    III.16, IV.02, IV.04, V.03,
    V.04
jaundice   I.08, IV.02
low birth weight   I.06, I.07,
    III.06, III.11, III.13, IV.01,
    V.04, VI.02, VI.07
malaria   I.06
medication   I.02, I.03, I.07, I.08,
    I.09, II.05, II.08, II.09, II.10,
    IV.01, IV.05
menstruation   I.07, IV.05
mental retardation   I.02, I.05
prematurity   III.11, VI.08
radiation therapy   I.01
rapid eye movements   (REMS)
    III.07
respiratory distress   I.05, III.02,
    III.09, III.10, III.12, V.03, V.04
schizophrenia   IV.05
septicemia   I.05, I.06
sleep cycle   III.07
still births   III.02, IV.01, IV.05,
    V.01
sucking behavior   I.04, I.06,
    VI.05
sweating mechanism   III.13
synergistic effects   I.01
syphilis   I.06, III.04, V.02
teratogenic effects   I.02, I.03,
    II.01, II.02, II.04, II.06,
    IV.02
tetanus   I.06
thrombophlebitis   I.05, III.02
toxemia   III.02, III.04, V.02
venereal disease   I.05, I.07, II.09,
    III.04
withdrawal symptoms   I.05, I.06,
    I.07, I.08, I.09, III.01, III.02,
    III.09, III.13, IV.01, IV.02, IV.03,
    IV.04, V.01, V.03, V.04, VI.01,
    VI.02, VI.05, VI.06